KU-525-632

HAIRSTYLE FILE

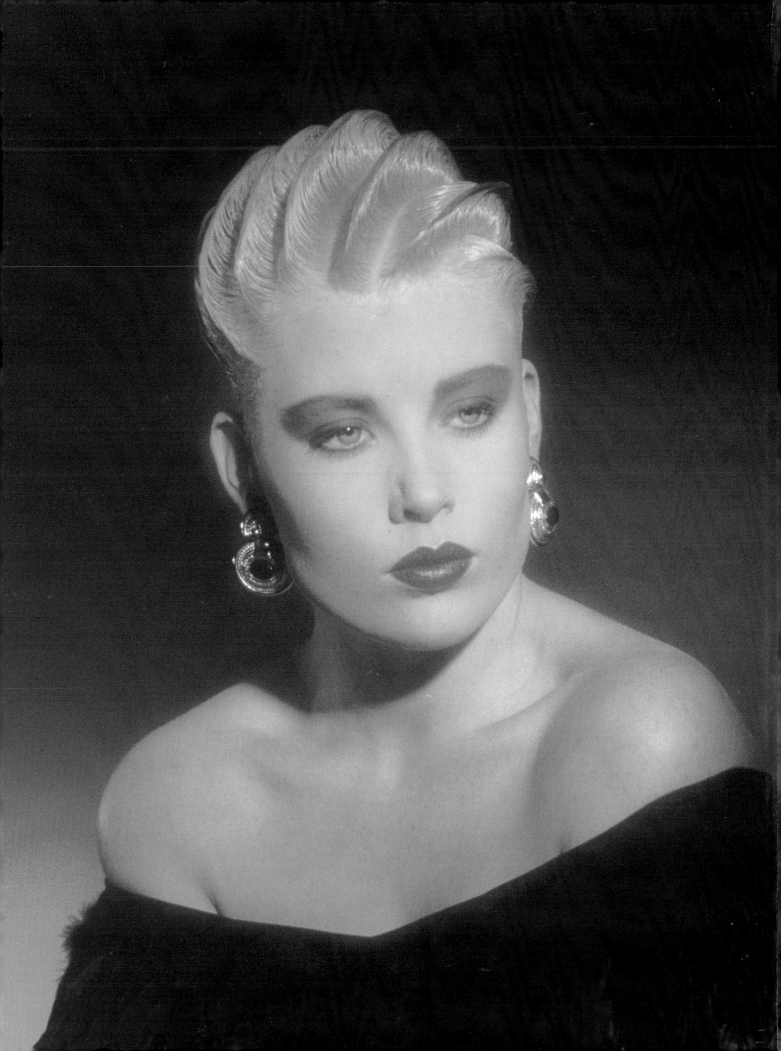

HAIRSTYLE FILE

Jacki Wadeson

WITHDRAW

Quantum
Books

646724 WAD
106229

A QUANTUM BOOK

This book is produced by
Quantum Publishing Ltd.
6 Blundell Street
London N7 9BH

Copyright ©MCMXC
Quintet Publishing Limited.

This edition printed 2003

All rights reserved.
This book is protected by copyright. No part of it may be
reproduced, stored in a retrieval system, or transmitted in
any form or by any means, without the prior permission
in writing of the Publisher, nor be otherwise circulated in
any form of binding or cover other than that in which it
is published and without a similar condition including
this condition being imposed on the subsequent
publisher.

ISBN 1-86160-676-1

QUMHSF

Typeset in Great Britain by
Central Southern Typesetters, Eastbourne
Manufactured in Hong Kong by
Regent Publishing Services Limited
Printed in China by
Leefung-Asco Printers Limited

Contents

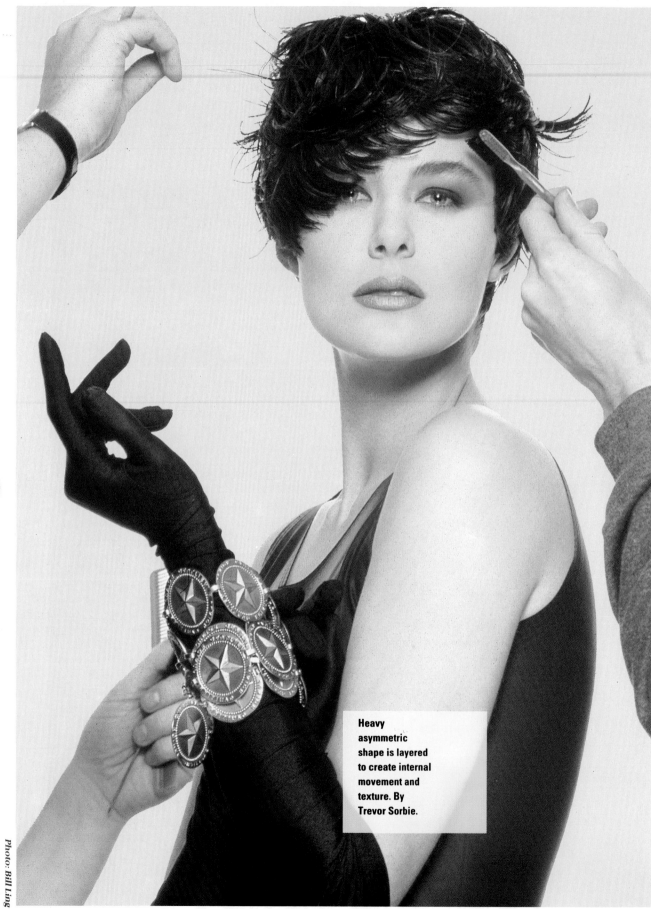

Heavy asymmetric shape is layered to create internal movement and texture. By Trevor Sorbie.

Photo: Bill Ling

Introduction

Hair is an exciting and extravagant medium that has always played a unique part in the way we look.

Austere styles have reflected times of war and hardship whilst flamboyant coiffures have been popular in times of plenty. Sculptors work with clay, artists work with oils but to hairdressers, hair is the ideal creative medium. Modern styling products have meant that it is now possible to do virtually anything with hair.

Hairdressers have always taken inspiration from couturiers but it wasn't until Raymond 'Teasy Weasy' brought hairstyling into the home with the first television hairdressing shows in the 50s that some of the mystery was taken out of the art of dressing hair.

After Raymond came Vidal Sassoon with his cut and blow-dry styles. These freed women from the earlier hard backcombed rigid looks and introduced them to a whole new hairdressing concept. Next came Trevor Sorbie with his visionary cuts and techniques including 'The Wedge', 'The Chop', 'Wolfman' and 'The Scrunch'. This revolution in hairdressing meant the end of the weekly salon visit for a 'wash and set'. Women wanted to be able to style their hair at home in the minimum of time with the minimum of fuss.

The most important change in hairdressing this century has been the discarding of the idea that we must all blindly follow what fashion dictates. It is now acceptable to wear a style that suits you, to take the best of the new techniques and tailor it to your hair and lifestyle.

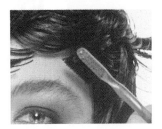

By all means take direction from the fashion statements shown in glossy magazines but don't be a slave to the scissors. The craft of hairstyling is now a fully appreciated part of the fashion industry, and the profession is enjoying a renewed acknowledgement that styling is an art form.

This book aims to take you through a plethora of beautiful styles and from the many pictures you are certain to find something that is just right for you. We explain how to choose your style, dry your style and then walk out in style. Featured here you will find the very best of international hair artistry – so if you want to be a cut above the rest just take a leaf from this book of styling magic . . . .

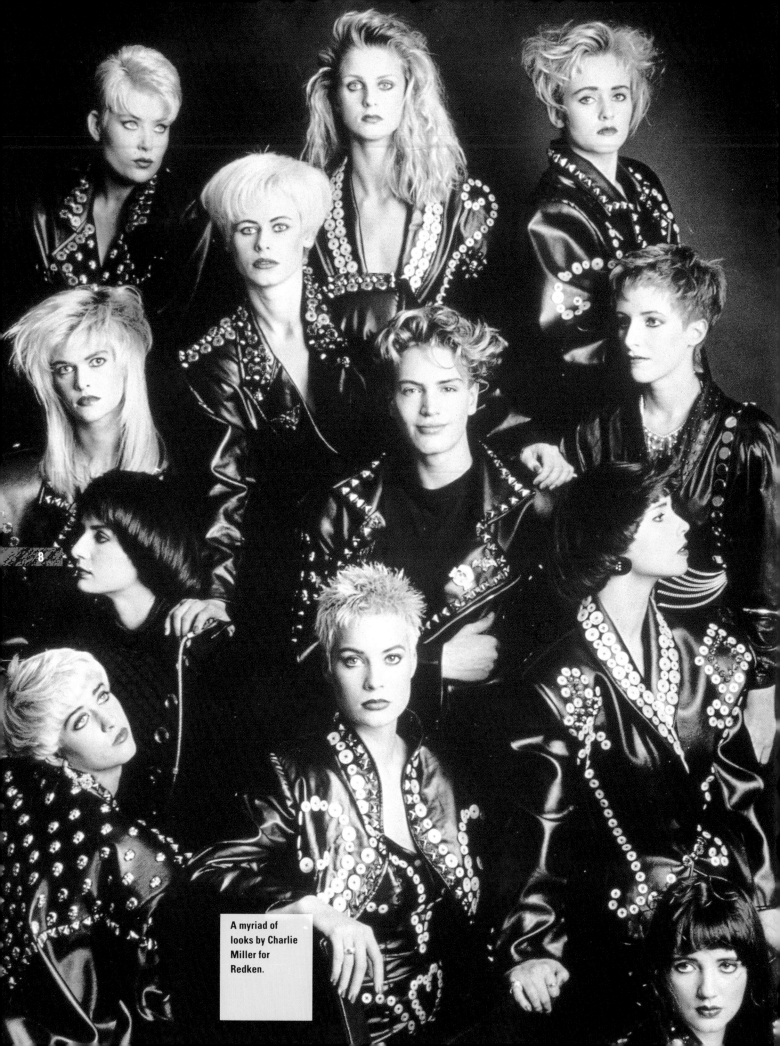

A myriad of looks by Charlie Miller for Redken.

Choosing a hairstyle

Modern hair reflects the easy mood of fashion and beauty. Your hair should complement your clothes and make-up but more importantly it should suit your personality. Nevertheless your lifestyle, hair type and texture, and face shape all play a part in the decision on the right style for you. Do you have the time and patience to cope with a style that needs complex care? Does your job demand neat, short or tied-back hair? Would you be better to choose a shaggy cut that needs little attention? Can you afford costly re-touching of an all over colour change?

KNOW YOUR HAIR TYPE

Thin or fine straight hair is best cut into a textured short style, or softly permed to give additional volume.

Medium textured and straight hair is very adaptable. If hair is in super condition a bob is ideal. Perming is also perfect for a full, curly look.

Fine curly hair needs precision cutting to keep it under control.

Thin, wispy hair is difficult to grow long and is often better styled shorter.

Thick and strong hair usually has a mind of its own. A mid-length cut is probably easiest to handle. Excess frizziness can be brought under control by combing with a wide toothed comb and dampening with water to re-set curls.

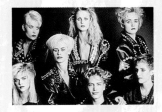

COLOUR

If you want a colour change try and choose a shade that suits your skin tone and eyes. One or two shades either side of your natural colour is best. There are several options:

Permanent The colour penetrates the hair shaft and is with you until it grows out.

Semi–permanent The colour will wash out within about six weeks.

Temporary colourants 'Wash'in, 'wash' out colours – ideal for a quick boost and special occasions.

Highlights Fine streaks of colour that aim to give a sun-kissed appearance are ideal for fair hair.

Lowlights Fine streaks of red or light brown tones to warm and lift the natural colour are ideal for brunettes.

PERMS

These don't necessarily mean curls, they can also be used to add extra body and volume. The variations on the perming theme are:

Root Perms These add lift to the first ½in (1cm) of hair.

Body-perms These give soft waves and volume.

Weave Perms These give a tousled effect.

Multi–textured perms The hair is permed on a combination of small and large rods to create a natural effect.

Spiral perms Longer hair is wound on to sticks or rods to give a corkscrew type curl.

RECOGNIZE YOUR FACE SHAPE

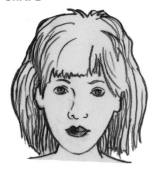

A pear-shaped face has a wide forehead, narrow chin area and small cheekbones. Choose a hair style with volume between the ears and shoulders. Avoid short crops and hair tied back in a ponytail.

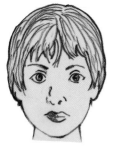

An oval-shaped face is wide near the temples narrowing down towards the chin. This is considered a near-perfect shape and means you can choose practically any style you fancy.

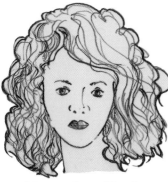

A heart–shaped face has a wide forehead and narrow chin. It looks super with a shaggy hairstyle with lots of volume.

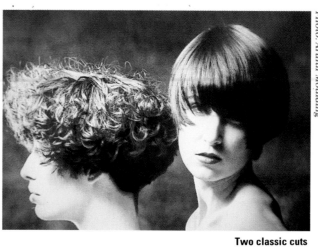

Photo: Arthur Moulding

A round face shape needs to be given an illusion of slimness. To do this choose a short style with waves and soft movement rather than a halo of curls. Centre partings and full fringes should be avoided.

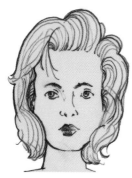

A square face has strong angular lines. Avoid very short styles as they can appear rather harsh. Instead try chin length looks with softness and texture. Accentuating the cheekbones with a drawn back style and fullness at the back of head can look stunning.

Two classic cuts with emphasis on front sections. Curly hair permed to give width, with deep copper tones applied for added interest. Straight hair cut to fall forward to frame the face. Block colour gives a healthy appearance. By Gregory Cazaly.

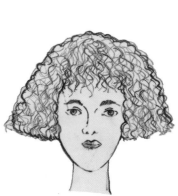

A long and thin face should not be accentuated by wearing hair hanging straight. Choose a style with softness and plenty of width. A bob is the perfect choice.

Three dramatic short styles. By Franklin Massahood at Morris Masterclass.

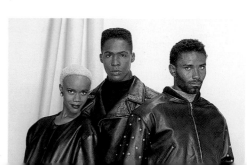

SPECIFIC PROBLEMS

Prominent nose Incorporate softness into your style.

Pointed chin Style hair with width at the jawline.

Low forehead Choose a wispy rather than a full fringe.

High forehead Disguise with tiny tendrils of curls.

Receding or flabby chin Select a style that's just below the chin level and has waves or curls.

Uneven hairline A feathery fringe will conceal this problem.

Widow's peak Here the hair growth in the centre of the forehead is lower than in the temple areas. To maximize the effect you should take the hair in the reverse direction to the growth. This gives the impression of a natural wave.

Cow's lick This is where on the forehead or neck the hair grows backwards and forwards at the same time. Clever cutting can re-distribute the weight and go some way to solving this problem.

Glasses Try and choose your frame style and hair to complement each other. Large specs could spoil a neat, feathery cut and conversely very fine frames could be swamped if you wear a large voluminous style. Remember to take your glasses to the hairdressers when having a restyle so that you can take the shape into consideration when deciding on the overall effect.

A GOOD CUT

The basis of any style is a good cut and without this investment all the styling aids in the world won't enable you to achieve lasting results. A short precision cut needs trimming every four weeks, a longer style every 6–8 weeks. Many different cutting techniques are used.

Blunt cutting or scissor-under-comb is used for developing strong outline shapes. Often this is followed by point tapering where the scissor points are clipped into the hair to thin sections and reduce weight.

Graduating means developing weight along a specific line taking into account the natural hair growth patterns and movement.

Texturizing means chipping into ends to create texture in specific areas to build up or remove weight.

Razor cutting is used to create softness and internal movement to any cut. It is either used on its own or in conjuction with scissors.

Layering removes weight and heaviness from hair.

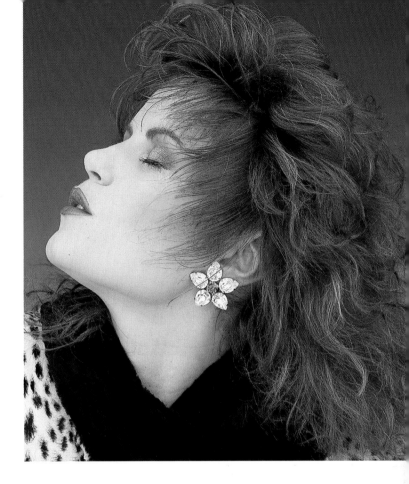

Layered, longer hair permed for softness. By Fields.

PROBLEMS

Dandruff This is where the natural process of the shedding of skin cells has for some reason got out of hand. The precise cause of dandruff remains a mystery but some experts believe it is the result of bad diet or illness, others that it's fungal infection. Dandruff should not be confused with a very dry scalp.

How to treat First make sure you are eating a healthy diet with plenty of whole grains, fresh fruit and vegetables. Cut down on fats, sugars and refined carbohydrates. Then try to increase the blood supply to the hair follicles by giving yourself a gentle scalp massage. Press your fingertips into your scalp at the sides of your head, and, keeping them in place, rotate them in small circles. The idea is to gently move the scalp, not the fingers. After about 30 seconds move to another part of your head and repeat until you have treated your entire scalp.

Avoid harsh 'anti-dandruff' shampoos, which can over-dry the scalp. Instead wash daily with a very mild, organic shampoo – this will help to control the greasiness and remove the loose flakes of skin. Every week moisturize the scalp with a rich conditioning treatment. If the problem persists consult your doctor or a trichologist. They will be able to recommend a special shampoo containing selenium which works as an anti-fungal agent.

Greasy hair This can be due to a hormonal imbalance; a diet too high in fatty foods; washing too often; or sometimes because the scalp has larger oil glands than normal.

How to treat Change to a healthy diet and try to reduce over-stimulating the scalp by washing hair less often. Use an oil-free shampoo every three days and avoid over-brushing or combing.

Dry hair This can be identified quickly by its dull, lack-lustre appearance. This is often the result of excessive perming or colouring. However sometimes it can be because the scalp has fewer oil glands than normal.

How to treat Avoid the use of heated appliances and steer clear of perming or colouring for the immediate future. Limit washing to once every four days and use a high-quality conditioner. Brush hair with a bristle brush to spread the naturally produced oil gently down the hair shaft. For short term use, a spray-on shine conditioning product will give instant sheen and a healthy looking appearance.

Hair loss A certain amount of hair loss is normal but excessive loss can be caused by eczema, alopecia, stress or a change in hormone levels. It may be due to taking the pill or pregnancy, excess alcohol or nicotine or quite simply tying the hair back too harshly.

How to treat Change to a healthy diet and if the condition doesn't improve it is a good idea to consult your doctor.

As you can see with the many variations of hair type and problems, your choice of style is an individual decision. The way you dress your hair is one of the simplest forms of self-expression. If you are happy with your hair, you will feel and look good.

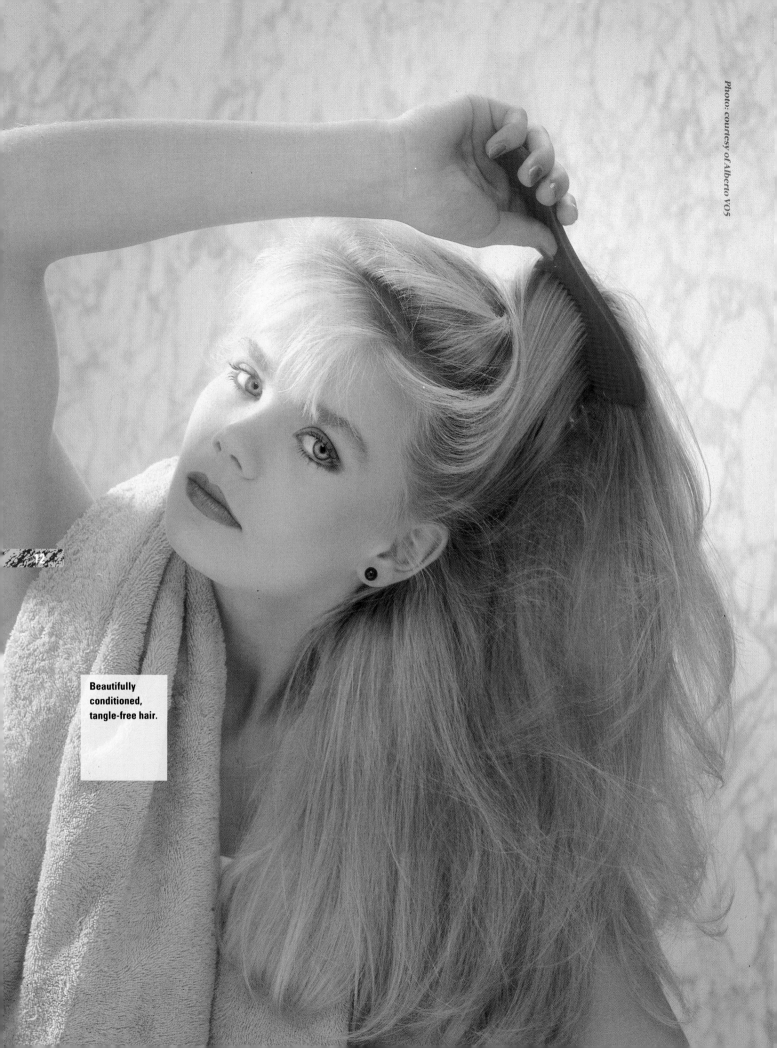

Beautifully conditioned, tangle-free hair.

Photo: courtesy of Alberto VO5

Styling aids

Hair oils were the first styling aids and developed to make curls last longer in humid atmospheres. These oils were produced by perfumiers from closely guarded recipes, handed down from generation to generation.

The waving iron was invented by Marcel Grateau in the eighteenth century. The technique of waving hair with the iron was called ondulation and it allowed natural looking movement to be formed. This method of applying waves took expert skills and proficient hairdressers were much in demand to produce waves *à la Marcel*.

Advances in chemistry and technology mean that we now have a wide selection of styling aids to transform hair whilst maintaining its condition.

SHAMPOOS

The object of shampoo is to cleanse the hair without stripping it of natural oils leaving it supple, tangle-free, glossy and full-of-body. Choose a shampoo that is formulated to suit your hair type. *Normal* hair needs a balanced cleanser; *dry* hair needs gentle cleansing and *greasy* hair requires deep cleansing.

Experiment with trial sizes of shampoos to find products that suit you. Remember always to rinse hair very thoroughly after shampooing to avoid any residue build-up. Also, be aware that the condition of your hair changes all the time depending on your health, chemical treatments and the weather. Products that are perfect for you at one point in time may need to be changed to allow for these variations.

If you suffer from dandruff, beware of strong anti-dandruff shampoos. Try an organic product first and if the problem persists consult your doctor or a trichologist.

CONDITIONERS

Conditioners are formulated to be used after shampooing to smooth down uneven cuticles. They work by coating each hair with a fine layer of oil which serves to make hair more manageable. *Normal* hair needs a balanced conditioner, *dry* hair needs deep conditioning whilst *greasy* hair needs a light conditioner. You can't build up condition on your hair – you need to re-apply conditioner every time you wash to maintain shine and manageability. Leave the product on for the time stated – neither longer and nor shorter – to work properly.

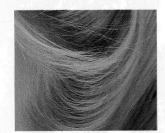

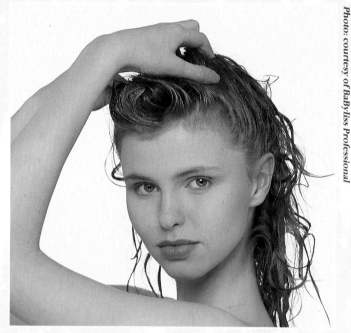

Photo: courtesy of BaByliss Professional

Treat your hair to an intensive conditioning treatment at least once a week.

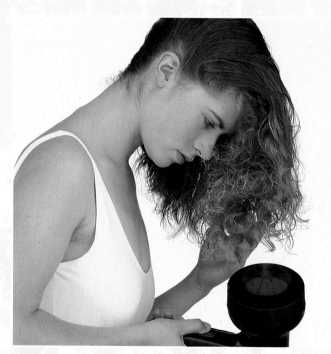

Photo: courtesy of BaByliss Professional

A softly, scrunched effect is easily created with an infra-dryer.

INTENSIVE CONDITIONING

Intensive conditioning products contain ingredients that are formulated to nourish the hair shaft of extra dry or damaged hair. They seal in the natural moisture and help to prevent further damage.

Most of these creams or waxes should be applied generously to the hair and left for five to ten minutes before rinsing out. For badly damaged hair the treatment effect can be intensified by leaving the product on for ten to twenty minutes and wrapping the hair in plastic cling wrap. *Do* follow the directions supplied with the product you choose.

STYLING PRODUCTS

There is such a wide variety of products available that it is sometimes difficult to know which one you should choose to get the desired result. In general, all the products are resin-based and aim to coat the hair and help hold it in place. Remember, don't use too much and apply the product to your hair, not your scalp, where it could cause irritation.

Forming cream is an opaque soft wax. Dab a little on to dry hair. Use to tame flyaway hair. Designed for thick or fine straight hair for which normal wax is too heavy.

Gel looks like jelly and usually comes in a tub or tube. Apply sparingly with your fingers to dry or damp hair. *Use* to create strong, spiky looks and root lift. Ideal for curl separation and more structured styles.

Professional tip Re-voluminize already gelled hair by running wet fingers through, against

Photo: courtesy of Silvikrin Active Care

the finished direction, before arranging.

Gel spray is an extra strong fixing product. Spray all over for maximum control. *Use* to give hold and lift and keep hair in place all day long.

Glaze is a runny gel usually sold in bottles. Pour a small amount into your hands, rub palms together, then stroke through wet or dry hair. *Use* to give a strong hold and support. It is ideal for sculptured styles, and perfect for sleeking down any frizzy ends on long bobs.

Hair spray is a glaze which comes in a aerosol or pump and is designed to control hair. *Use* to give

A shoulder-length bob is beautifully conditioned and then scrunch-dried.

Photo: courtesy of BaByliss Professional

support and lasting power to your style. It can be used on all hair types and styles to give extra body, volume and control. Good products should control without stickiness or flaking. If you want your hair to go back but

Place a handful of hair into a diffuser dish – the 'lifters' help to separate and ruffle hair as it dries.

it is intent on flopping forward, hold your head back and spray round hair line. Put the dryer right into the roots to make it stay in place.

Mousse Mousse is a foamy setting product that is used on damp hair or between washes on dry hair. Squeeze out a small amount on to hand and stroke through hair. *Use* to achieve natural-looking body and texture. Ideal for fine, flyaway hair, because it adds volume as well

Photos: courtesy of BaByliss Care Plus.

as getting rid of static. Use extra hold mousse on very fine hair to give root lift. Excellent for scrunch-drying. Mousse also boosts curls in permed or naturally wavy hair.

Don't over-mousse short hair an egg sized amount is enough. Too much doesn't add to the effect, it has the opposite effect by weighing it down.

Professional tip Re-activate curls or de-frizz over-dried hair by coating hands with mousse then working through the outer layers of the hair.

Restructurant is a spray conditioner. Apply quite liberally to dry, badly conditioned hair. *Use* to

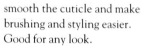

Drying a
sculptured look
with a diffuser.

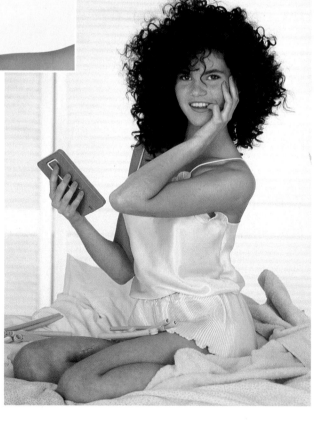

Smooth out kinks by spritzing lightly with water and blow-drying on a low speed and low heat setting.

smooth the cuticle and make brushing and styling easier. Good for any look.

Spray-on shine is a conditioning spray. Spritz over dry hair after styling. *Use* to give instant gloss. It is superb on naturally frizzy hair leaving it more controllable and less dry on the ends.

Spritz is a spray-on setting lotion. Apply to wet or dry hair. *Use* to make curls last longer. It adds height to short cuts if used on root area and gives body to long hair.

Adding lots of curl using hot sticks.

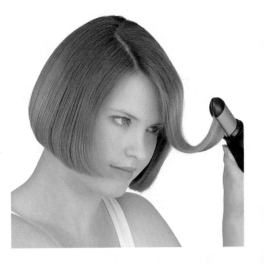

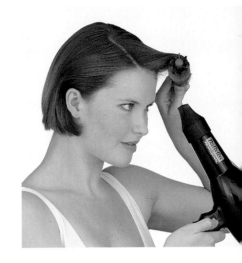

Adding body and curl by blow-drying hair with a circular brush using a styling nozzle on the dryer.

Small sections of hair are straightened and curved.

Wax is a thick, solid grease that is best used on dry hair. Simply warm a *little* wax in the palms of the hands, transfer to fingertips and apply to the hair, shaping and defining as you go. *Use* to achieve spikes, points, a sleek, flat look or simply add extra shape and sheen to waves, curls, bobs and ponytails. Styling wax also helps control static and put control back into just washed, flyaway hair. It will also help to counteract the after perm 'frizzies'.

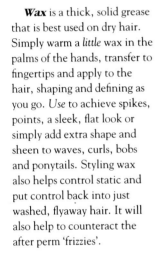

A sleek and smooth blow-dried look.

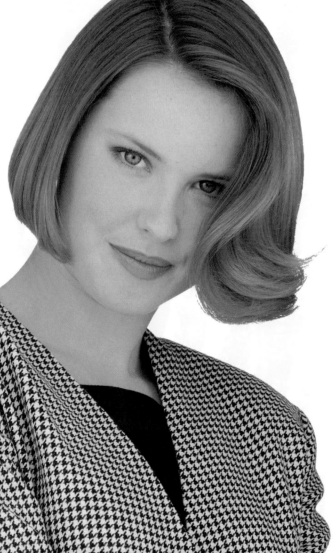

HAIRSTYLING APPLIANCES

The range of electrical equipment available for use at home means that you can achieve a truly professional look every day of the year.

Crimping irons are flat irons with undulating plates of varying degrees. Hair must be previously straightened either by blow-drying or using flat irons, then the crimper is used to create instant waves and styling effects.

Curling tongs create curl, control, shape and body. Tongs can also be used to create a temporary curly effect producing a mass of ringlets or spiral curls. They are available in two varieties: *slim* for curling shorter hair and creating wispy ringlets; and *standard* for longer length hair.

Professional tip Perfect tonging takes practice but once the technique is mastered you can create a galaxy of looks. The best way to tong is to slide the tongs into the hair close to the roots and then wind the section of hair around the barrel. Make sure that the ends of hair are neatly tucked in, close the level and hold for a few

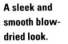

seconds before releasing the curl. Repeat as necessary to achieve style.

Diffusers fit on to the nozzle of the dryer to give a gentler heat without the blow. This way of drying is especially effective on permed or naturally curly hair. The low air-flow is also good for fine, flyaway hair. The best diffusers have 'lifters' or 'prongs' which separate and ruffle the hair as it dries.

Professional tip To create a structured look on short hair towel dry hair and apply gel. Style into place using a comb and fingers then hold the diffuser still, drying a section at a time. For a casual naturally-curly effect on long hair, you should towel dry hair and apply mousse. Place sections of hair into the dish of the diffuser as it dries. To finish, rake the curls gently with the fingers.

Flat irons come in a variety of shapes: large and

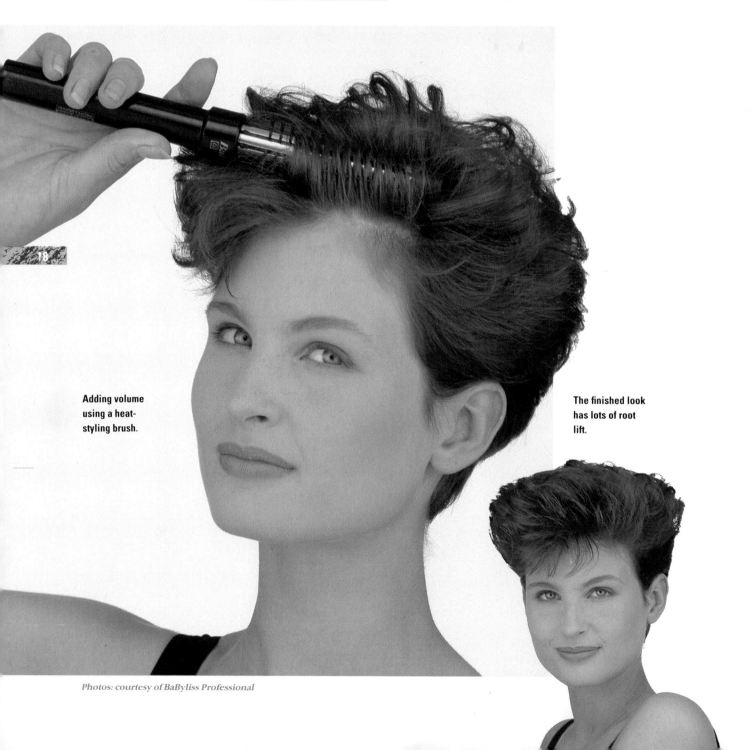

18

Adding volume using a heat-styling brush.

The finished look has lots of root lift.

Photos: courtesy of BaByliss Professional

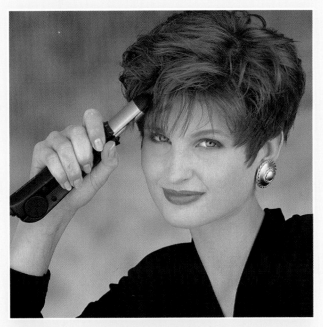

Use a
straightener,
close to the
roots, to create
lift, texture and
movement.

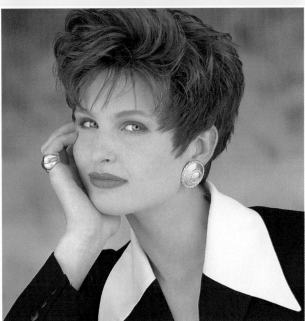

A neat and
controlled style.

flat or smaller and finer. The object is to smooth and finish the hair. They are designed literally to iron-out stubborn ends and give a glossy, smooth finish. The larger irons are for long straight locks. The small irons are for shorter styles to give straightness plus a softening curve at the end. To use, work section by section and slanting at the roots, slide the iron down the hair shaft, turning ends under if desired.

Flexibrushes with steam are styling brushes with soft, flexible bristles. Incorporated in the brush is a water reservoir which when heated produces jets of steam designed to 'set' curls. They are ideal for creating soft, gentle curls and waves on longer hair.

Hairdryers can be used to dry any style. Choose a 'professional' model which is designed and built to the exact requirements for salon use. These powerful dryers give up to 1,500 hours of drying time as against the average consumer dryer lasting for approximately 300–400 hours. Choose one with an additional narrow styling nozzle for a precision-controlled air-stream. In addition, make sure the dryer has multiple heat and speed combinations with a cold (not cool) button for 'setting' the hair. Also ensure that the dryer has a removable air filter so it can be easily cleaned. *Professional tip* Lower settings are much kinder to the hair and give much more control.

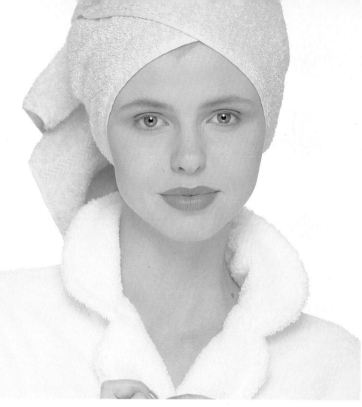

Photo: courtesy of Silvikrin

When using a deep action conditioner, wrap your hair in a warm towel and leave for 20 minutes.

Always remember to use a shampoo formulated to suit your hair type.

Heat-styling brushes are brushes combined with a heated rod. *Use* to control unruly hair or to add body and volume to straight hair. Simply wind small sections of hair round brush and hold for a few seconds. Leave to cool then brush or scrunch into place.

Professional tip: If you pull each section forward before winding, the curl will spring back on itself to give style extra fullness.

Heated rollers are solid and heat up to a controlled setting. *Use* to give instant lift and bounce to a style. Ideal after blow-drying and before putting hair up as it gives additional body.

Hot brushes are particularly good for adding volume, body and bounce. They come in all shapes and sizes, and are great for shorter styles and for adding finishing touches to blow-dried hair.

Professional tip: A slim tong will achieve a tight curl whereas a fatter tong will produce a looser curl.

For extra fullness, pull each section of hair firmly forward before curling. Each curl will pull back on itself, giving your style extra body and fullness.

Hot sticks and benders are smooth rods that are heated up before use. *Use* on dry or slightly damp hair, with mousse or gel. Perfect for instant permed looks or just body and waves. To use, simply section hair and wind around the hot stick, leaving for five to ten minutes before removing and dressing out hair. For a more dramatic effect take small sections of hair and twist before winding on to the rods.

Infra-dryers are a relatively new concept that intensify the benefits of diffuser drying. The combination of diffuser and infra-red lamp, dries the hair with gentle heat rays rather than hot air. They are perfect for naturally curly, permed or short, structured cuts. This method of drying gives an even result without over-drying the ends.

DRYING TECHNIQUES

Blow-drying involves using a dryer and brush. Roll hair around a circular brush getting it tight at the roots.

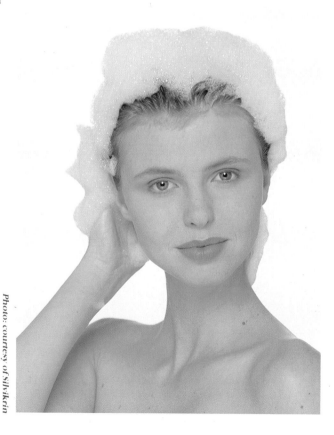

Photo: courtesy of Silvikrin

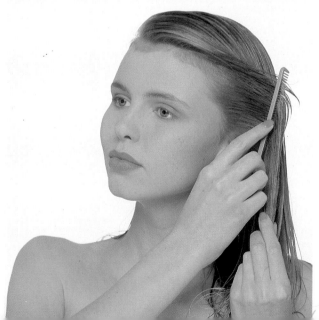

Photo: courtesy of Silvikrin

Attach a directional nozzle to the dryer and aim the dryer straight at the roots. Rotate the brush gently as you dry each section. Let each area cool for 30 seconds before removing brush. Work through the head, section by section, in the same way.

Gel drying is best for shorter styles. Coat fingers with gel and run through hair to distribute evenly. For maximum movement, with height and width, lift hair and aim dryer at the roots. Make sure the ends are dry but where you're holding the hair nearer the roots, should be left damp. This gives lift with a texturized outline.

Natural finger-drying creates soft waves. Apply mousse or gel and comb hair into desired style. Allow to dry naturally, tousling and loosening the hair as it dries. Finish with a little wax.

Scrunching is screwing up small bunches of hair in the palm of your hand, aiming the nozzle into the centre of the palm for 15–20 seconds, and letting the hair cool for a further 20 seconds to set the scrunch in. This works best on damp, moussed hair to produce voluminous, tousled styles. A similar, more controlled effect is achieved by using a diffuser for scrunching. The action of the diffuser spreads the air-flow, lifting the hair at the roots. With your free hand lift, ruffle and lightly scrunch the hair as you gently rotate the diffuser against the hair.

Professional tip: Big scrunched styles need drying with the head tilted downwards. Rake fingers through for maximum lift. When the hair is dry throw your head up again and arrange as desired.

Remember to distribute mousse evenly to the entire head.

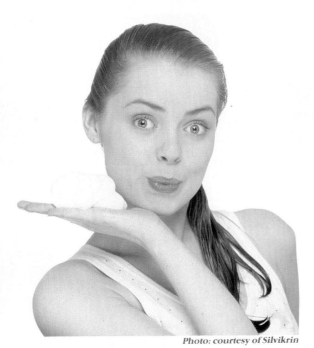

Photo: courtesy of Silvikrin

left **Comb conditioner through the hair to help remove tangles and knots.**

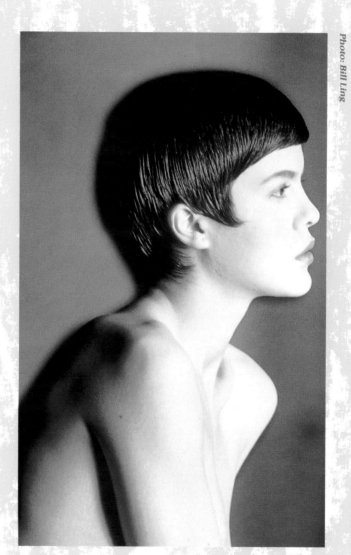

Photo: Bill Ling

A strong
geometric shape
achieved by
layering the hair
throughout. By
Trevor Sorbie.

Short styles

When hairdressing maestro, Antoine, cut Coco Chanel's hair into a bob in the 1920s he started a hairdressing revolution. Up until then long hair was the fashion with short styles considered not only distasteful but indecent! Women who dared to wear their hair short were a target of ridicule. In order to achieve the look, without the cut, women resorted to pinning up their hair in a variety of ways to resemble a bob. However, the austerity of post-war Britain affected the whole social strata. Soon women were doing men's jobs and needed hairstyles that were easy-to-manage. Hence the trail was blazed for new trends in hairstyling.

These days neat, short hair is an acceptable part of being a modern woman . . . and is softer, more natural, more versatile than ever. High-fashion cuts have heavy fringes and internal layering. To encourage movement and texture a cutting technique called 'slicing' is often used.

The look can be curly or straight, all-over blunt or softly layered to frame the face. Lift and volume can be achieved using mousses and gels. A variety of drying techniques make styling easy. Finger-drying for soft waves; scrunch-drying for a tousled look; blow-drying for a more positive line and natural drying for the ultimate wash 'n' wear.

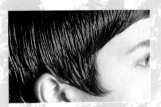

Short hair should always be in tip-top condition and this is achieved by regular cutting and conditioning. Colour plays an important part on shorter hair. For dark heads, blackberry, redcurrant and blueberry tones create vibrant shine and texture. For blonde hair, shades are cooler and more natural . . . paler hues to pure red tones. For brunettes, burnished lights can be added for depth and intensity. Wash-in, wash-out colours are the easiest way to give your hair that subtle difference without having the problem of re-growth. Most temporary colours have built-in conditioners which also add extra shine. Highlights are always popular but forget 'blonde streaks'. Today's techniques aim to give a sunkissed look. Dappled effects can be achieved using slices of rich, warm brown or burgundy.

Permanent colour can be a big step – and a big commitment. Before embarking on this type of colour change you must find the perfect shade. Perms are ideal for giving short hair added body, movement and, of course, curl. Short back and sides doesn't have to mean drop on top. Fine, limp hair can be given added volume and thickness; unruly, heavy hair can be more easily controlled and previously permed hair can be given a new lease of life by lifting and styling from the roots. A gentle perm on the crown will give height and volume.

Styles displayed on the following pages show how versatile short cuts can be.

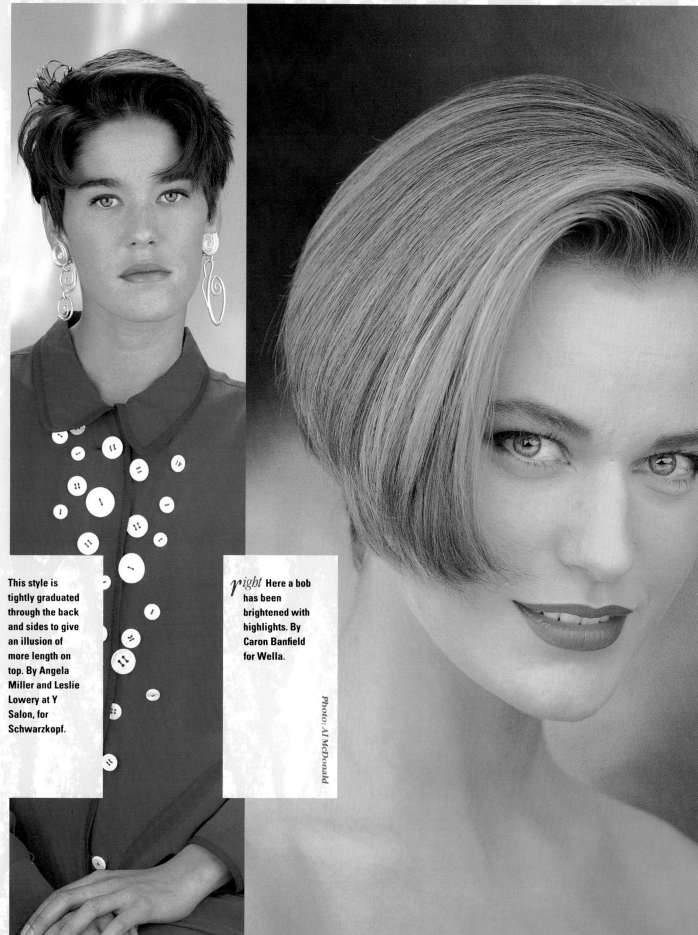

This style is tightly graduated through the back and sides to give an illusion of more length on top. By Angela Miller and Leslie Lowery at Y Salon, for Schwarzkopf.

right Here a bob has been brightened with highlights. By Caron Banfield for Wella.

Photo: Al McDonald

Photo: Martin Evening

Photo: Anthony Mascolo

*l*eft A 'shattered' bob dressed using mousse which gives control and support for this pretty look. By Toni & Guy.

*r*ight This elegant style is coloured with an intensive gold. By Wendy Sadd for Clynol Hair.

Photo: Eammon McCabe

*l*eft Hair is coloured using a dark mahogany. By Jeni for Clynol Hair.

*l*eft The hair is lifted by scrunching with gel and pinning up sides with combs. By Jeni for Clynol Hair.

Photo: Pete Underwood

Photo: Pete Underwood

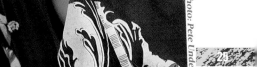

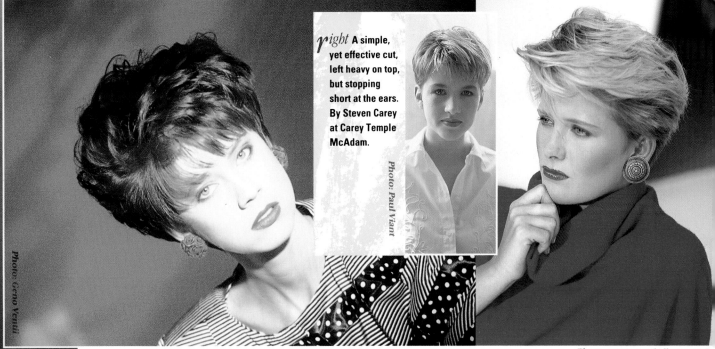

*r*ight A simple, yet effective cut, left heavy on top, but stopping short at the ears. By Steven Carey at Carey Temple McAdam.

Photo: Paul Viant

Photo: Geno Ventii

Photo: courtesy of Alberto VO5

*a*bove A glamorous long, crop, coloured golden brown, is finger-dried to encourage plenty of height at the crown. By Nando at Geno Ventii for Schwarzkopf.

*a*bove An easy-to-manage style full of body and shine.

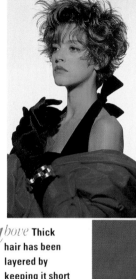

a^{bove} **Thick hair has been layered by keeping it short at the nape and longer through the front. By Nicky Clarke at John Frieda.**

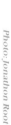

b^{elow} **A sharp effect is achieved here by straightening the hair using a directional nozzle on a dryer. By Gary Hooker at Saks for Clynol Hair.**

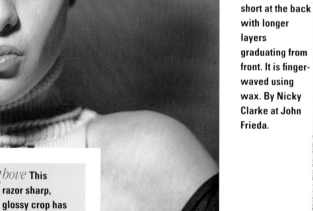

Photo: Raphael

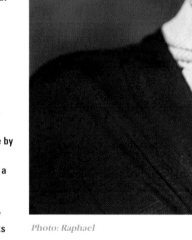

Photo: Jonathon Root

a^{bove} **This razor sharp, glossy crop has a graduated fringe. By David Field at Fields.**

b^{elow} **This style is coloured mahogany and blow-dried to add definition. By Jason Rushton at Unique for Clynol Hair.**

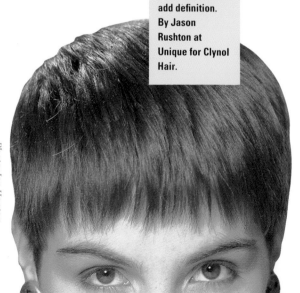

Photo: Ian Hooten

a^{bove} **The hair is cropped short at the back with longer layers graduating from front. It is finger-waved using wax. By Nicky Clarke at John Frieda.**

b^{elow} **A brilliant blonde, slither cut throughout and finger-dried directionally. By Cobella for Schwarzkopf.**

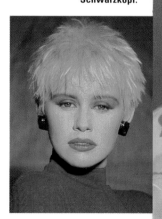

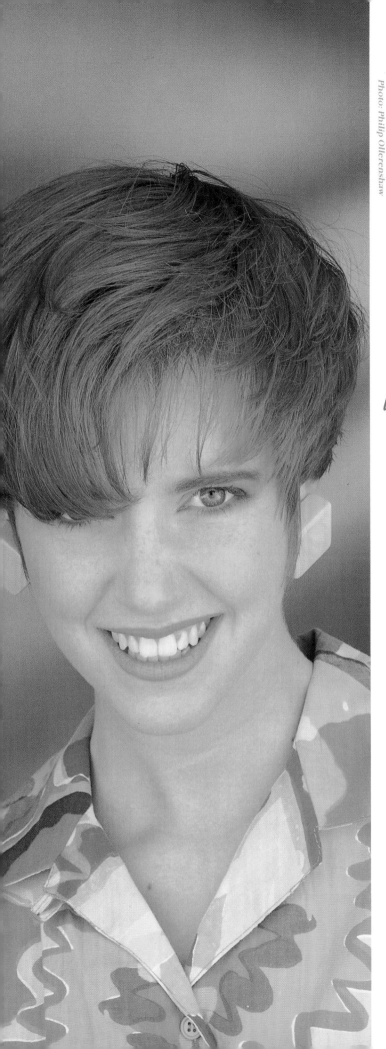

Photo: Philip Ollerenshaw

right **An easy-to-wear beach style – simply combed back with gel. By Simon Grigg at Philipsharon for Wella.**

Photo: Patrick Jackson

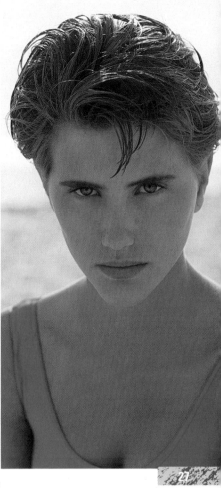

left **An asymmetric cut on a brilliant redhead. By Steve Ryding at Steve Ryding Trimmers Group for Wella.**

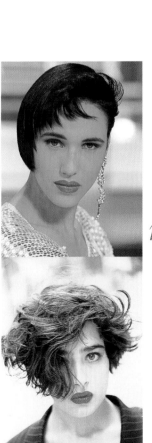

left **A beautiful glossy evening look with kiss-curl fringe. By Ellis Helen for Clairol Professional.**

right **This heavy bob is conditioned to perfection and dressed forward from the crown. By Guy Kremer for Schwarzkopf.**

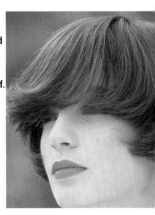

left **Here the movement and texture of the hair is created with slice-cutting. By Toni & Guy.**

Photo: Anthony Mascolo

below **This short, graduated bob is dried forwards with a blow-dryer. By Gary Hooker at Saks for Clynol Hair.**

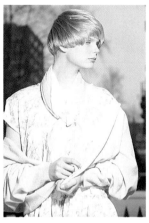

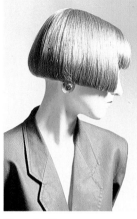

left **A chic, classic bob cut in a straight line. It sweeps softly forward to caress the cheekbone, with a heavy fringe to accentuate the shape. By Steven Carey at Carey Temple McAdam.**

right **A geometric cap of shiny smooth hair. By Rita Rusk International.**

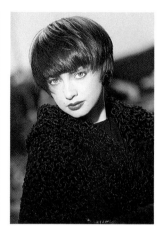

Photo: Melissa Halstead

Photo: Ian Forster

Photo: Mac

Photo: Bill Ling

right **These curls were dressed using an extra strong styling spray. By Karen Banfield for Clynol Hair.**

28

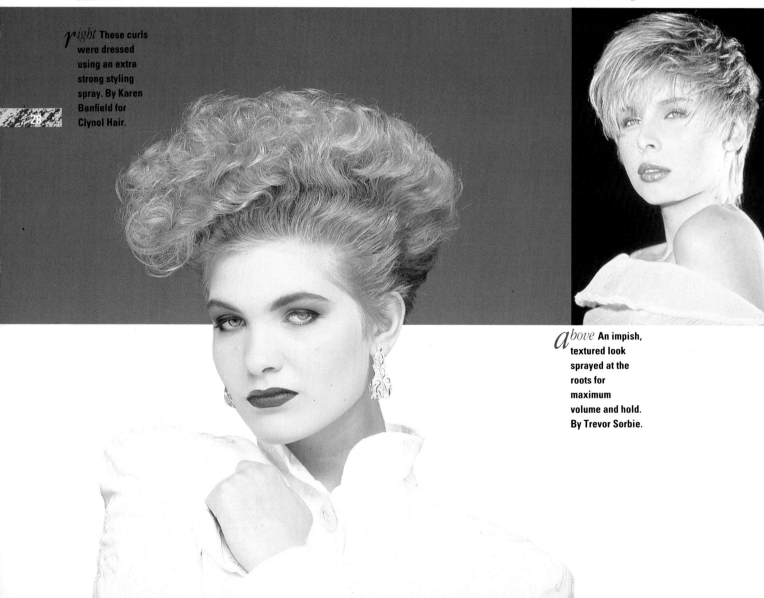

above **An impish, textured look sprayed at the roots for maximum volume and hold. By Trevor Sorbie.**

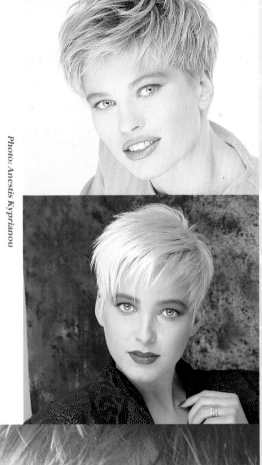

Photo: Anestis Kyprianou

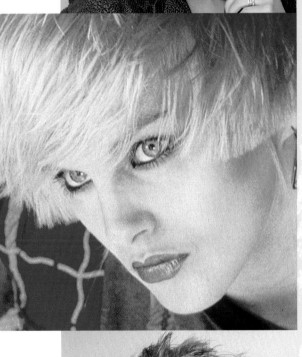

Photo: David Darling

Photo: Gary Lyons

left The hair is cut short with longer layers through the top. It was dried using a forward directional movement to achieve a soft finish. By Beverly at Cobella for Schwarzkopf.

left This style is very short at the nape and slither cut throughout the sides and top to give a soft, textured appearance. By Anita at Cobella for Schwarzkopf.

below A strong, very short cropped look. By Anthony Mascolo at Toni & Guy.

Photo: Anthony Mascolo

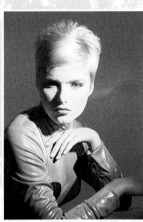

below A short, layered bob. By Michael Gerrard at Barnard, Wilmslow for Wella.

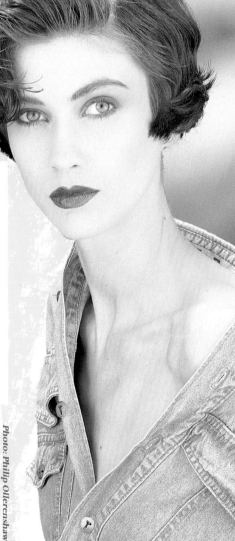

left Here naturally straight hair is cut into a blunt bob with graduated layers. By Karen Wood at Melvin & Friends.

left This shattered short cut has a broken fringe. By Paul Mitchell.

Photo: Philip Ollerenshaw

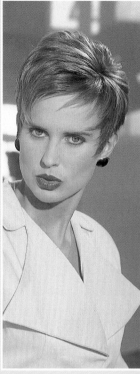

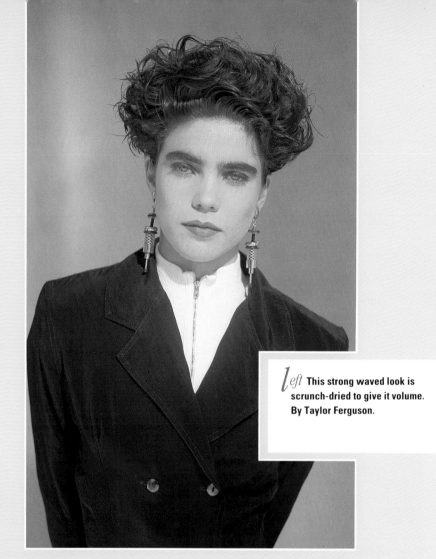

above **A cheeky elfin cut. By Andrew Collinge.**

below **This fine hair is cut short through sides and back, and left longer on top. By Michelle Flower at Level.**

left **This strong waved look is scrunch-dried to give it volume. By Taylor Ferguson.**

right **The hair is razor cut and dressed forwards encouraging height at the crown. By Andrew Collinge.**

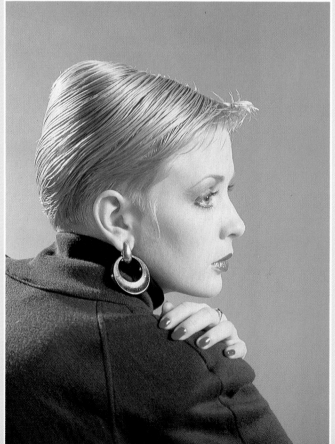

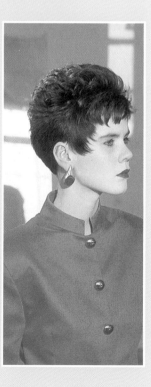

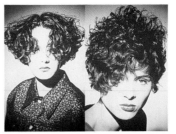

*r*ight **Both of these styles are graduated to create curl and movement. By Toni & Guy.**

Photos: Anthony Mascolo

*b*elow **These sophisticated soft curls are created by scrunch-drying. By Taylor Ferguson.**

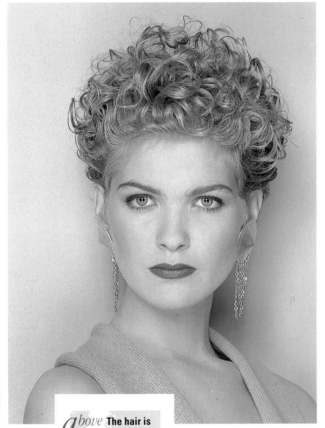

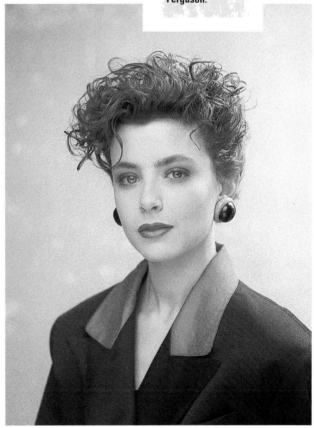

31

Photo: Bill Ling

*a*bove **The hair is brushed back and styled using the fingers to push the waves into place. By Beverly Kyprianou at Cobella for Schwarzkopf.**

Photo: courtesy of Alberto VO5

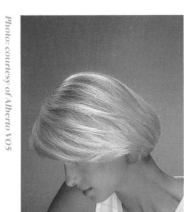

*l*eft **A sleek, club-cut blonde bob, highlighted to accentuate style.**

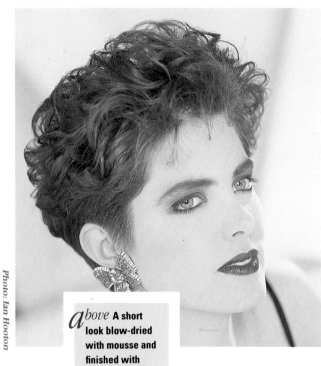

Photo: Ian Hooton

Photo: Leslie Lowery

above **A short look blow-dried with mousse and finished with hairspray. By Kim Le-Neveu at Boiler House for Clynol Hair.**

right **A striking crop with razored sides. By Wendy Sadd for Clynol Hair.**

above **A soft, internally layered bob dressed with mousse for fullness. By Angela Miller at Y Salon.**

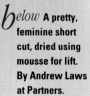

left **A sophisticated finger-waved gelled look. By Paul Mitchell.**

below **A pretty, feminine short cut, dried using mousse for lift. By Andrew Laws at Partners.**

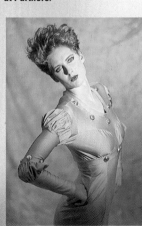

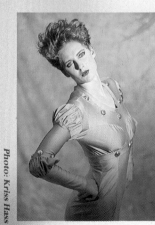

Photo: Kriss Hass

Photo: Eammon McCabe

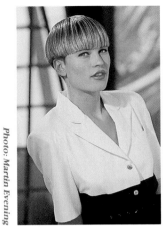
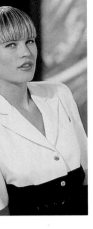

Photo: Martin Evening

left **A 20s bob, with a geometric strong line. The solid fringe is slightly clipped for texture. By Partners for Schwarzkopf.**

above **A short, layered cut slicked with wax and dressed into a side quiff. By Guy Kremer at French Connection.**

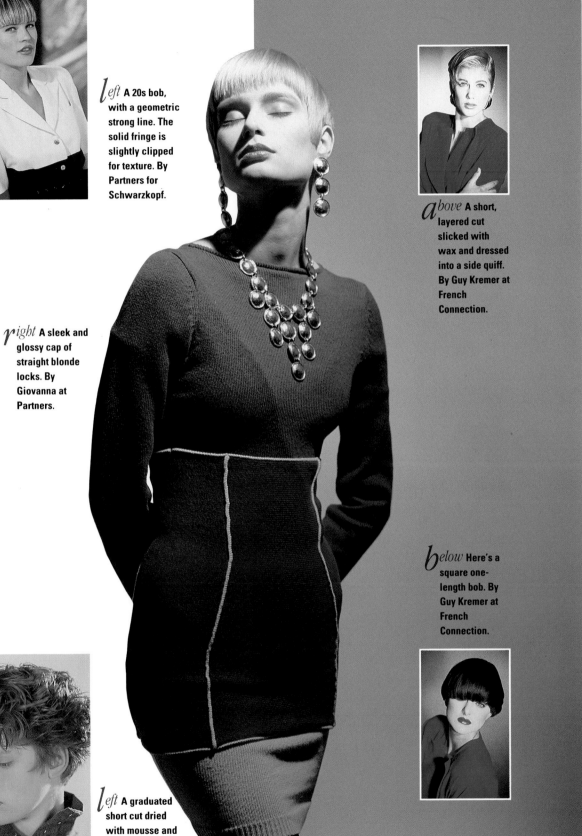

right **A sleek and glossy cap of straight blonde locks. By Giovanna at Partners.**

below **Here's a square one-length bob. By Guy Kremer at French Connection.**

left **A graduated short cut dried with mousse and finished with wax. By Fields.**

Photo: Keith Berry

Photo: Martin Evening

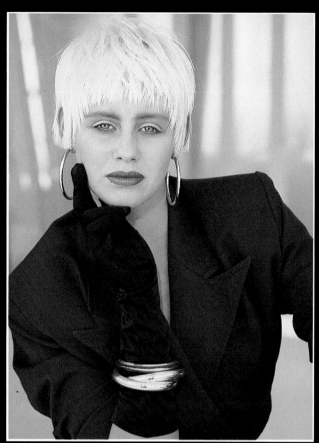

right **A square-shaped long crop, blow-dried using mousse and gel for shine and control. By Beverly Kyprianou at Cobella for Schwarzkopf.**

below **The looped fringe sections give interest to this neat cut. By Martin at French Connection.**

Photo: Paul Viant

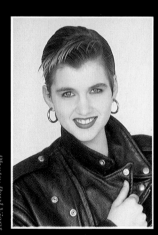

above **Here the fringe hair is gelled forward into a quiff to add interest. By Jo Seward for Carey Temple McAdam.**

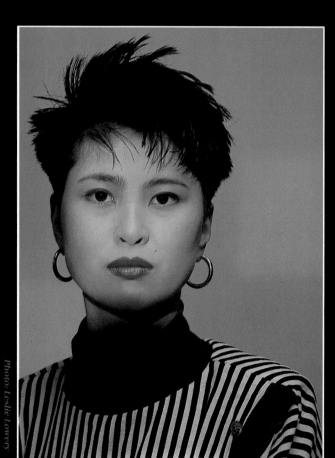

Photo: Leslie Lowery

left **This is a strong, chipped-in cut with a blue rinse to give it additional shine. By Angela Miller at Y Salon for Schwarzkopf.**

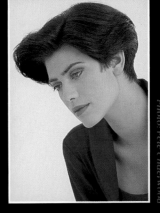

right The hair is coloured with a semi-permanent dark mahogany tint. By Jeni for Clynol Hair.

Photo: Pete Underwood

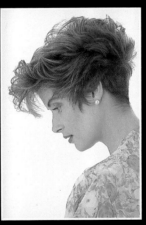

Photo: Pete Underwood

left Straight hair is permed for this soft, feminine look. By Jeni for Clynol Hair.

below This naturally curly hair is finger-waved at the roots and scrunched on top. By Taylor Ferguson for Schwarzkopf.

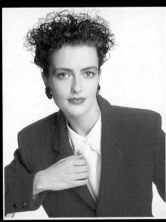

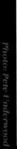

Photo: Pete Underwood

left Here a soft perm creates natural-looking waves. By Jeni for Clynol Hair.

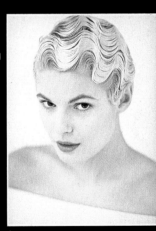

above Blonde hair is strongly finger-waved for this sophisticated style. By Paul Mitchell.

Photo: Pete Underwood

right This striking look is achieved by perming. By Jeni for Clynol Hair.

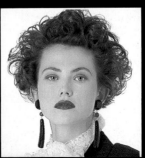

right The top hair is left long while the back is clippered. By Steven Carey at Carey Temple McAdam.

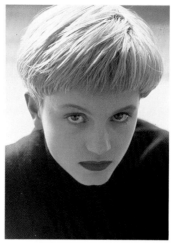

Photo: Ian Forster

below This stylish blonde crop is lightened using bleach. By Peter Baptist at John Gerard for Wella.

Photo: Philip Ollerenshaw

below A mass of glimmering auburn lights enhance this short look. By Carey Temple McAdam.

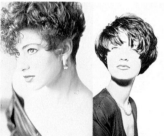

Photo: Ian Forster

Photo: Anestis Kyprianou

above Here, internal layering is left fairly long and heavy to increase volume through the sides. By Beverly at Cobella for Schwarzkopf.

right Colour gives additional lift with highlights. By Caron Banfield for Wella.

Photo: Al McDonald

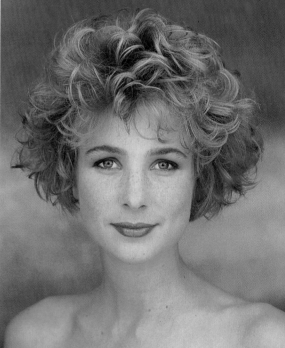

right Here a choppy, short look forms points around the face giving a broken line. By Ian Duncan at Partners for Schwarzkopf.

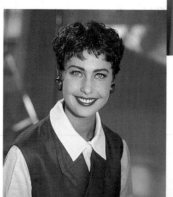

Photo: Martin Evening

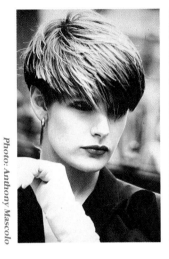

Photo: Anthony Mascolo

*l*eft Thick hair is cut into blunt layers and highlighted. By Toni & Guy.

*b*elow This basin shape was blow-dried using a round brush. By Stephen Wake at Level.

Photo: Colleen du Fay

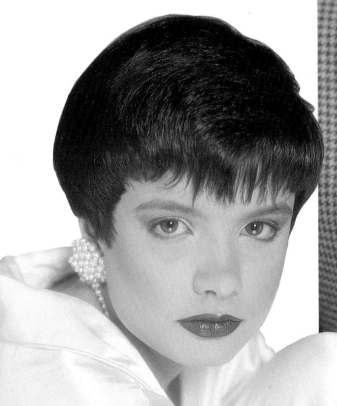

*a*bove This hair is finger-dried using wax for curl definition. By Taylor Ferguson for Schwarzkopf.

*r*ight Here a blonde highlighted bob is dressed forward from the crown. By Andrew Laws at Partners.

Photo: Kees Bass

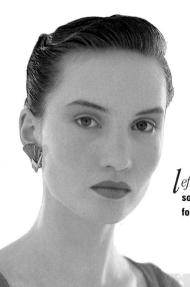

left The hair is coloured medium golden brown and softly waved using gel. By Richard Dalton at Claridges for Clairol Professional.

Photo: Stevie Buckle

Photo: Salvatore

right A shiny, short bob with blunt cut layering. By Christopher Dove at Sophisticut.

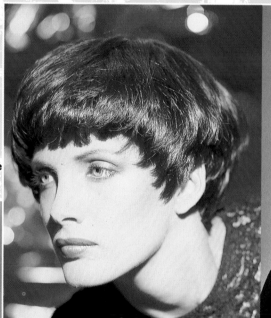

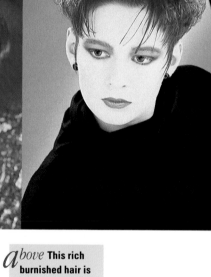

above This rich burnished hair is scrunch-dried using extra hold mousse. By Stevie Buckle for Wella.

left These sleek, slick waves are created with wet gel.

Photo: courtesy of Wella

left Here tightly permed hair is allowed to dry naturally.

Photo: courtesy of L'Oreal

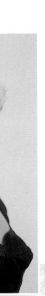

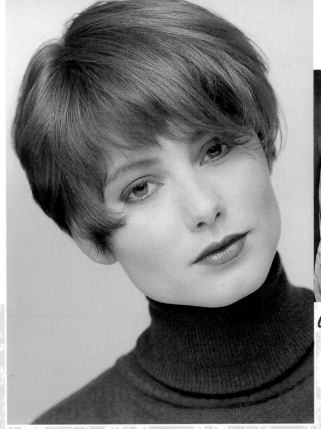

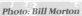

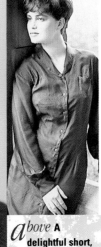

Photo: Kriss Hass

*a*bove This bleached blonde hair is strongly finger-waved. By Paul Mitchell.

*a*bove A warm, golden tone is achieved using a semi-permanent colour. By Ian of Scissors for Wella.

Photo: Bill Morton

*a*bove A delightful short, glossy cap of hair. By Ian Duncan at Partners.

*b*elow The hair is textured and feathered on to the face with a quiff at the side. By Stephen Wake at Level.

Photo: Colleen du Fay

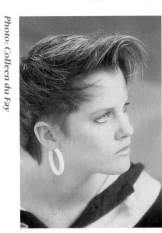

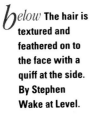

Photo: Peter Pfander

*l*eft A dramatic bob with gleaming auburn highlights. By Ian Duncan at Partners for Schwarzkopf.

*a*bove Here's a swinging cheek-length bob which is achieved by softly graduating the hair ends for gentle shape and movement. By Paul Edmonds for Schwarzkopf.

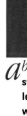

39

Photo: Kriss Hass

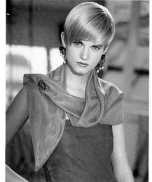

Photo: Martin Evening

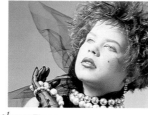

above These feminine curls are dried with a diffuser. By Fields.

above Here an asymmetric fringe is cut with a forward movement and graduated following the head shape at the back. By Ian Duncan at Partners for Schwarzkopf.

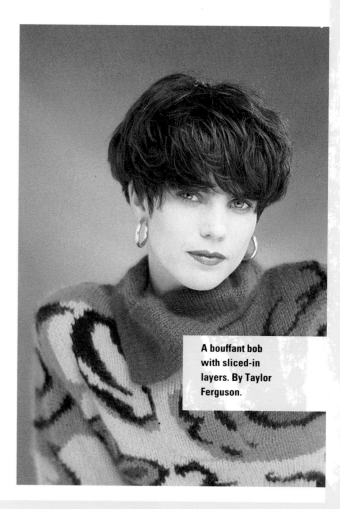

A bouffant bob with sliced-in layers. By Taylor Ferguson.

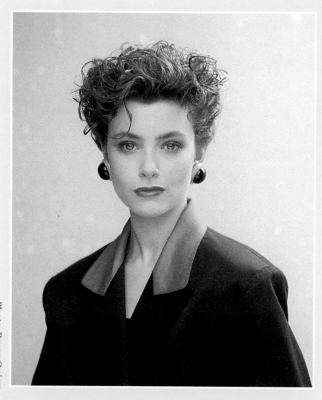

Photo: Bryan Quinn

right Curly, titian hair, styled using mousse to add texture. By Philip's Hair Studio for Clynol Hair.

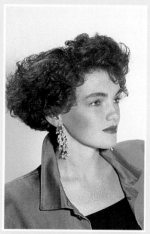

Photo: Chris Bishop

left Here the hair is swirl-dried to give movement and volume. By Taylor Ferguson for Schwarzkopf.

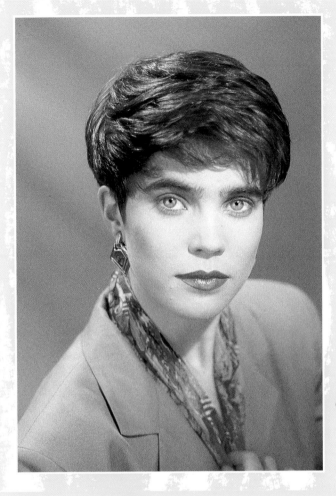

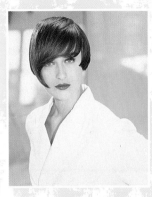

Photo: Martin Evening

right This balanced bob shape rounds towards the eyes with a larger section weave-cut for asymmetric eye detail. By Ian Duncan at Partners for Schwarzkopf.

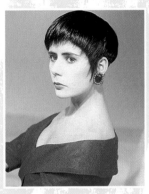

right A feather-cut fringe and sides give added impact to this style. By Taylor Ferguson for Schwarzkopf.

left This strong, internally-layered cut is dressed forwards. By Taylor Ferguson.

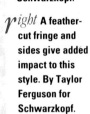

43

right The hair is permed for body then the back is gently graduated. By Avril at André Bernard.

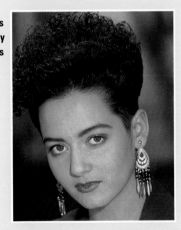

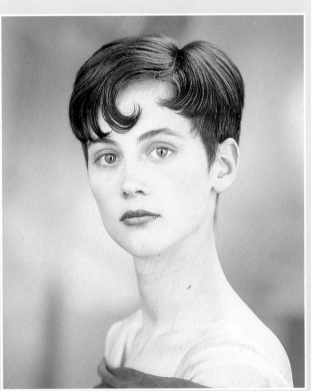

Photo: Martin Evening

right Golden lowlights give interest to this scrunch-dried style. By Terry Calvert at Clipso for Schwarzkopf.

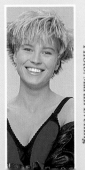

Photo: Martin Evening

above Here highlights in three shades – plum, mahogany and copper – give a burnished look. By Liz Edmonds for Schwarzkopf.

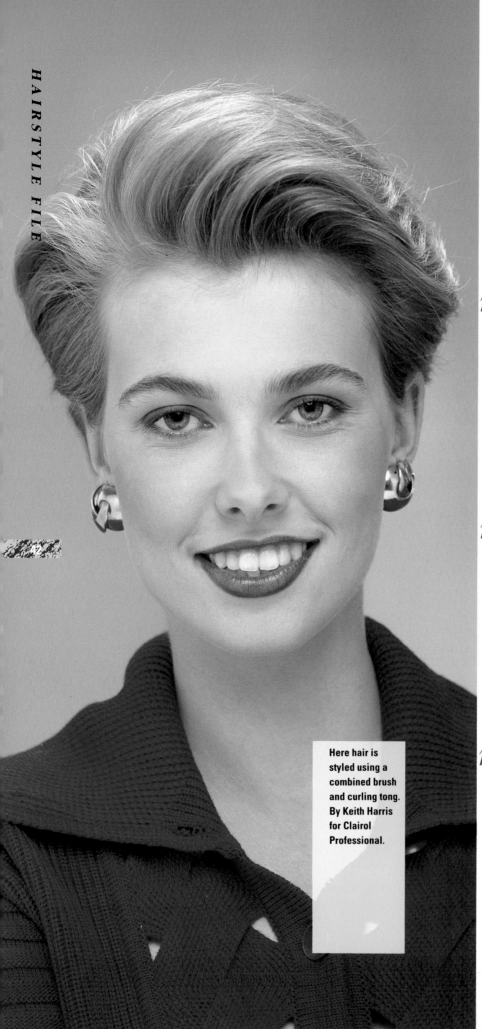

Here hair is styled using a combined brush and curling tong. By Keith Harris for Clairol Professional.

below **A stunning bleached blonde. By Taylor Ferguson for Schwarzkopf.**

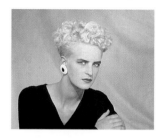

right **This is a bouncy perm, finger-dried with strong styling mousse. By Stephen Wake at Level for Schwarzkopf.**

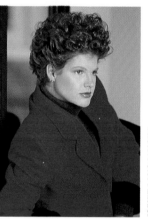

Photo: Peter Pfänder

right **This round-shaped bob has been cut using long layers to break up the texture and bring out the natural curl. By David Adams at Macmillan.**

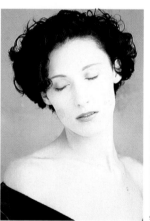

Photo: Arthur Moulding

right **This hair is cut into an urchin shape around the face and chopped into for texture. By Trevor Sorbie.**

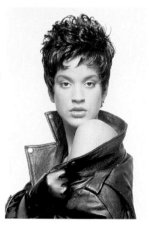

Photo: Bill Ling

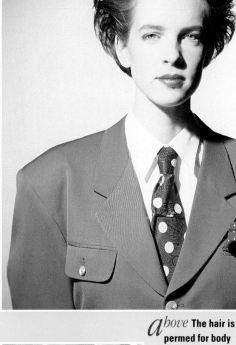

Photo: Liz McAuley

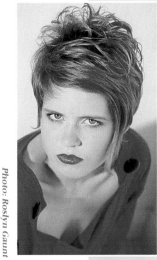

Photo: Roslyn Gaunt

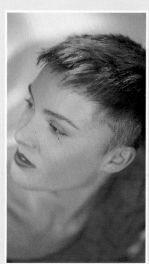

Photo: Eammon McCabe

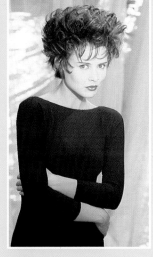

Photo: Martin Evening

*a*bove This style is razor-cut on the outside and blunt cut on the inside to give height at crown. By Alison White at Dom Migele.

*a*bove The hair is permed for body rather than curl and styled using mousse. By Louise Valentine-Lane for Clynol Hair.

*a*bove A pert style glistening with lights of strawberry blonde. By Wendy Sadd for Clynol Hair.

*r*ight The hair is root permed and teased into shape when still wet to give a softly gelled look. By Karen Banfield for Clynol Hair.

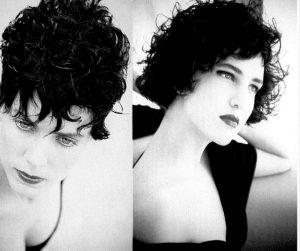

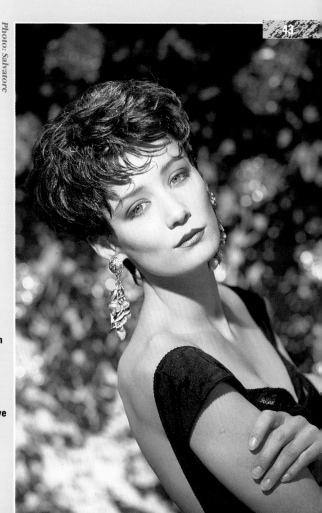

Photo: Salvatore

*l*eft Shattered outlines give a feminine freedom to these styles. By Toni & Guy.

*r*ight High-fashion creation is given lift and volume using mousse on the root area. By Christopher Dove at Sophisticut.

Photos: Anthony Mascolo

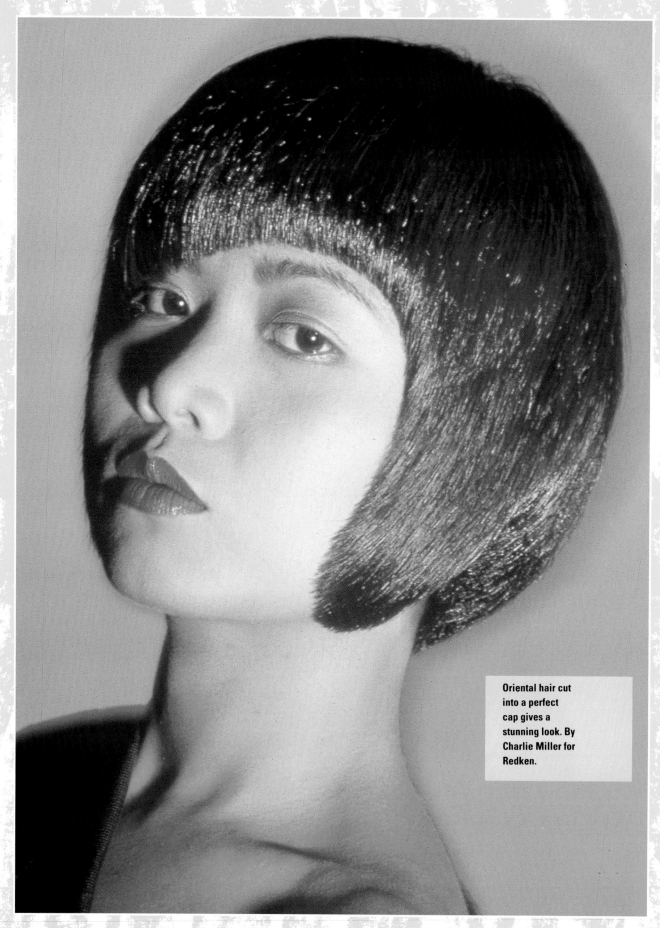

Oriental hair cut into a perfect cap gives a stunning look. By Charlie Miller for Redken.

Mid-length hair

During the early 30s women who had previously welcomed the short crop had tired of its uniformity. They

wanted something different but not a reversal to the long dressed styles of their ancestors. Marcel waving was still popular but it was the advent of the perm that made mid-length hair a fashionable proposition. Charles Nessler was the man who invented a fearsome looking machine that put curls into hair. After the First World War a new permanent wave method was found which was much simpler than Mr Nessler's huge machine. It was a chemical process that literally baked the curls into place. Women now demanded curly, tousled heads rather than small neat silhouettes.

Modern perms and techniques are a far cry from the first products and machines which were often used with disastrous results. The cosmetic discovery of pH balance led to the marketing of sophisticated perming solutions that are kinder to

hair and give predictable and efficient results.

The page-boy style – a sleek look with turned-in ends – was first popularized by Hollywood film star Greta Garbo and many variations on this theme are popular today.

Mid-length hair is perhaps the most versatile length. It can be worn straight and sleek, wavy or curly to give a variety of looks. If the nape hair is left longer it is possible to gel mid-length hair into a short ponytail and combs can be used to great effect by clasping side hair up and away from the face. One of the most important points to remember if you choose a mid-length bob is the importance of regular trimming. Split ends ruin a good line and the only solution is to snip them off. There is no product on the market that will repair hair that is damaged in this way.

Hair worn mid-length, especially in a long bob, needs to shine and glimmer in the light. If your hair lacks lustre it could be that the cuticle or outer layer has been damaged. The cuticles should be perfectly smooth and covered

in a natural secretion of oil. The hair shaft which is made up of overlapping layers will only reflect the light when it is smooth. The main reason for damaged cuticles is chemical treatments which literally have to lift the layers in order to penetrate the shaft. Use a conditioner to smooth down the cuticles and coat each hair with a fine layer of oil which will make it more manageable and help eliminate tangles. However, beware of over-conditioning as this can have the reverse effect making the hair dull and lank.

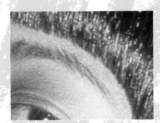

On the following pages you will find a galaxy of styles to suit every type of mid-length hair.

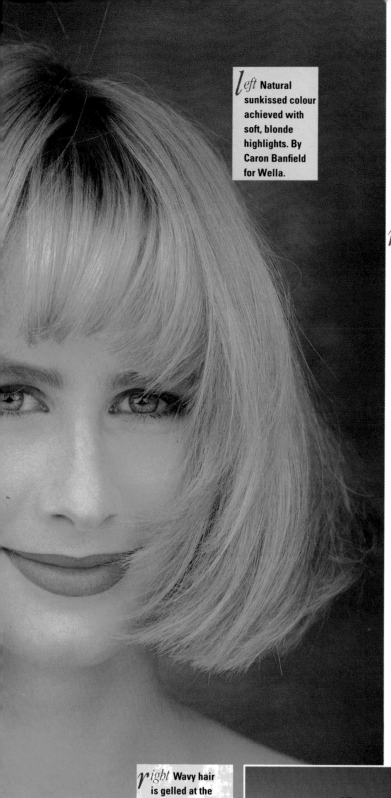

*l*eft Natural sunkissed colour achieved with soft, blonde highlights. By Caron Banfield for Wella.

*r*ight Permed to create sophisticated 30s waves. By Tony Connell at Worthington Hair for Wella.

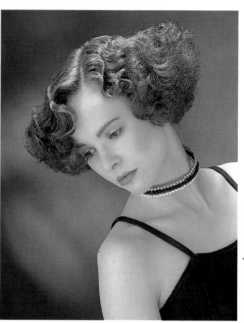

Photo: Philip Ollerenshaw

*l*eft Layered bob of soft, feminine curls. By Toni & Guy.

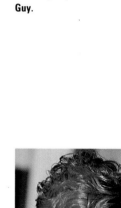

Photo: Anthony Mascolo

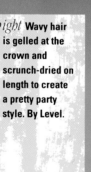

*a*bove This naturally wavy hair has been cut to remove weight at the back, but leaving length, height and width at the crown. By Ann-Marie Crighton at Dom Migele.

Photo: Roslyn Gaunt

*r*ight Wavy hair is gelled at the crown and scrunch-dried on length to create a pretty party style. By Level.

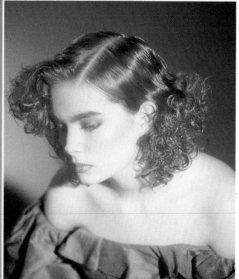

Photo: Al McDonald

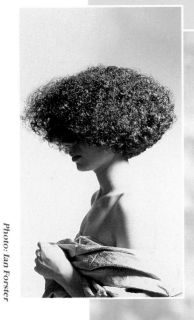

Photo: Ian Forster

*l*eft Afro hair cut into a round, almost circular bob shape. By Steven Carey at Carey Temple McAdam.

*r*ight A stunning brunette with a sleek, shiny bob. By Natalino Cargius at Don Giovanni for Wella.

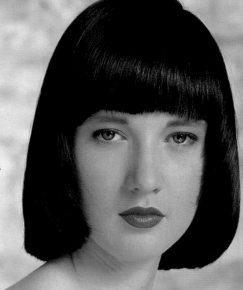

Photo: Chris Dawes

*r*ight This wild and free internally layered bob is scrunch-dried for volume. By Charlie Miller for Redken.

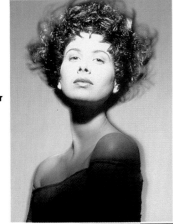

47

Photo: courtesy of Alberto VO5

*l*eft This fine blonde hair is cut into a neat bob and dressed to frame the face softly.

*r*ight A smart, one-length bob blow-dried to give lift at the roots. By Caron Banfield for Wella.

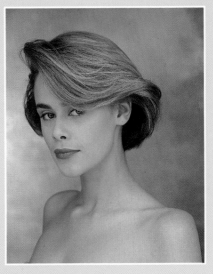

Photo: Al McDonald

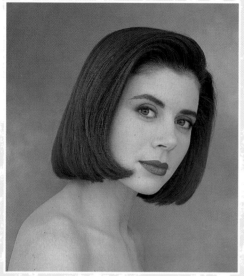

Photo: Al McDonald

left **Clever use of lowlights give this cut added panache. By Caron Banfield for Wella.**

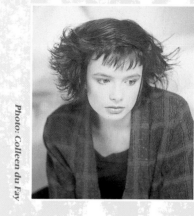

Photo: Colleen du Fay

left **A pert, ruffled cut with feathered fringe. By Level.**

right **A glamorous evening stunner with wispy fringe and longer tendrils dressed on to the neck. By Melvin Wood at Melvin & Friends.**

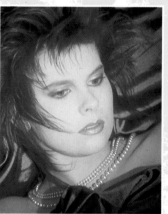

Photo: David Darling

left **Tongs or pin curls can be used to create tight curls. By Angela Miller at Y Salon.**

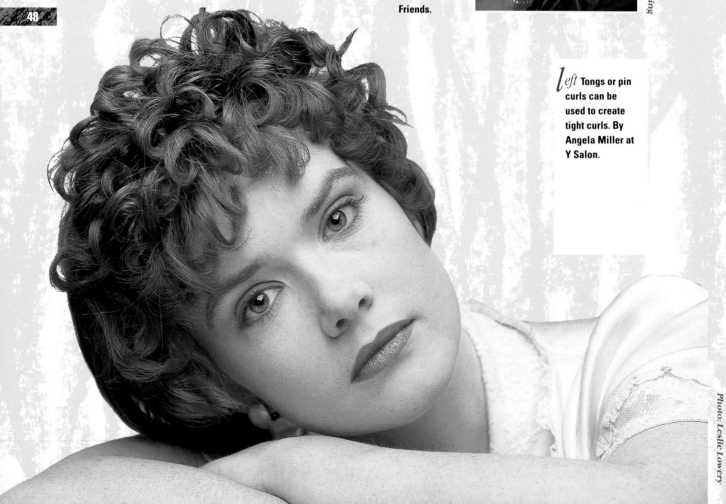

Photo: Leslie Lowery

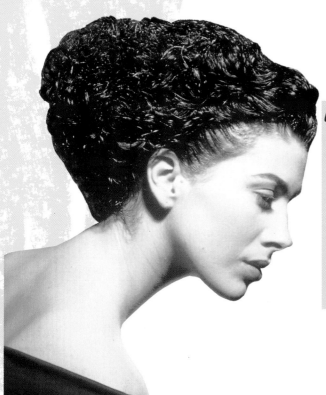

left Very curly hair swept up and away into a conical sphere. By Jason Miller for Redken.

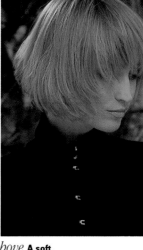

above A soft, tousled effect looks good on a blonde bob. Subtle layers create a face-framing shape. By Fields.

49

right Flick-ups can be blow-dried into place using a dryer and circular brush. By Stephen Wake at Level for Schwarzkopf.

below Naturally curly hair has been finger-waved then scrunch-dried with the head held forward to give added volume.

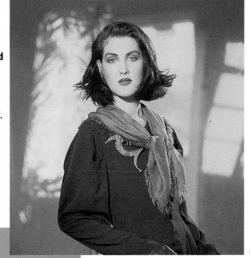

Photo: Martin Evening

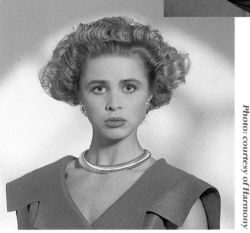

Photo: courtesy of Harmony

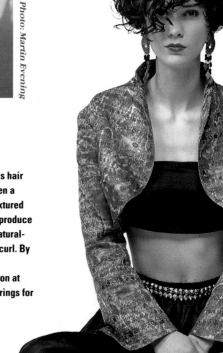

right This hair was given a multi-textured perm to produce a soft, natural-looking curl. By Alison Chesterton at Palm Springs for Zotos.

Photo: Bill Morton

right Thick hair is side parted and swept away from the face for this sophisticated look. By Charlie Miller for Redken.

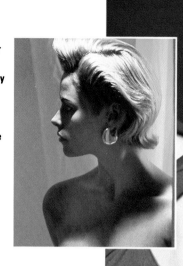

right A bleached blonde bombshell reminiscent of Marilyn Monroe. By Paul Mitchell.

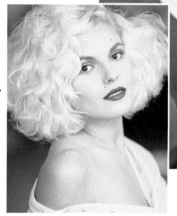

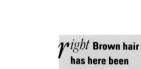

Photo: Graham Cooper

above This fine hair is permed using a combination of small and large rods to give maximum volume. By Alison Chesterton at Palm Springs.

right Brown hair has here been given a rich, gleaming sheen using a semi-permanent colour in jet black. By Ian at Scissors for Wella.

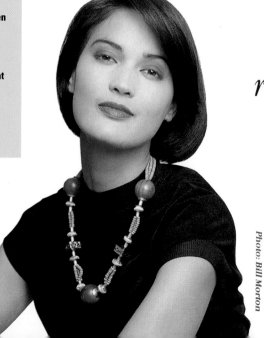

right This permed hair is scrunch-dried for all-over volume. By Mary D'Wit for Clynol Hair.

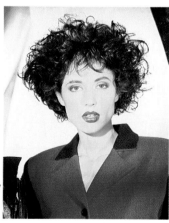

Photo: Martin Evening

Photo: Bill Morton

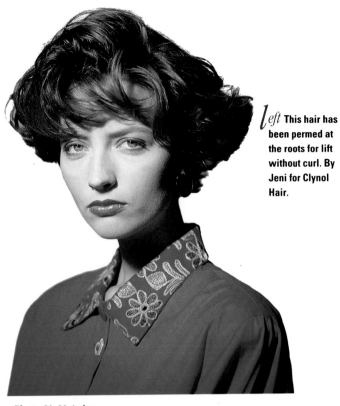

left This hair has been permed at the roots for lift without curl. By Jeni for Clynol Hair.

Photo: Liz McAuley

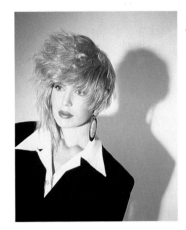

left Strawberry blonde with layered top and longer length graduated down the sides. By John Oliver for Schwarzkopf.

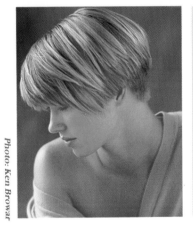

left Longer top layers give movement and a feeling of carefree chic. By Mod Hair, France for Schwarzkopf.

Photo: Ken Browar

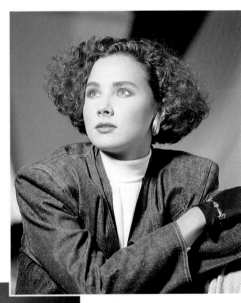

51

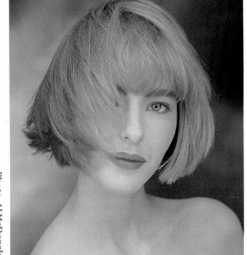

above Permed hair is finger-waved away from the face for this elegant style.

left A carefree bob with pale blonde natural-looking highlights. By Caron Banfield for Wella.

Photo: Al McDonald

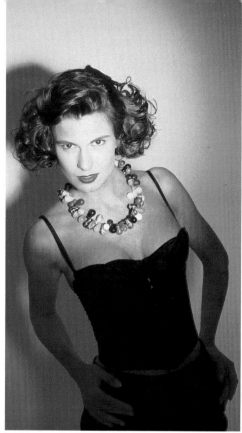

Photo: Bernd Nicholaisen

Photo: courtesy of Dimension Shampoo

right Height is achieved here by drying hair with the head held forward.

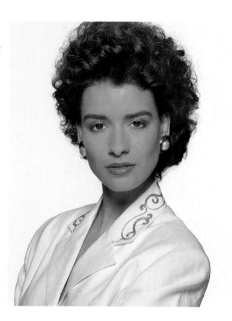

left This hair is coloured a beautiful burnished copper and finger-dried using wax for additional sheen. By Model Hair Artistic Team, Switzerland.

right A simple bob given width and height by blow-drying. By Philips Hair Studio.

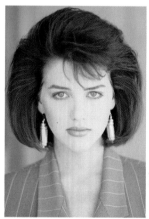

52

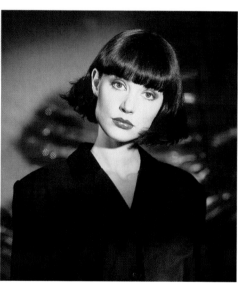

right A smooth bob needs regular intensive conditioning to keep the sheen and shine. By Karen Banfield for Clynol Hair.

Photo: Martin Evening

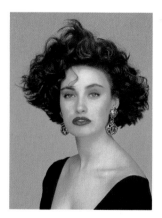

left Hair dried using the diffuser adaptor on a hand dryer in order to mould waves and curls into shape. By John Frieda.

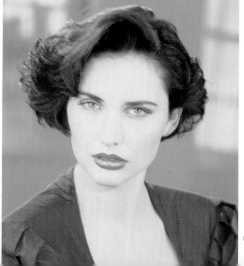

right Burnished red lights give added interest to this simple cut. By Edmonds for Schwarzkopf.

Photo: Martin Evening

Photo: Colleen du Fay

right This stunning creation contrasts straight hair against tumbling curls. By Stephen Wake at Level.

Photo: Arthur Moulding

right Here smoky blonde and silver blonde lights give lift and softness. By Stephen Wake at Level for Schwarzkopf.

left Flyaway hair was conditioned then cut into a square bob with a layered fringe. By Guy Kremer for Schwarzkopf.

Photo: Steven Henderson

A classic bob shape has been slightly graduated to encourage an outward movement at the ends. By Level.

Photo: Colleen du Fay

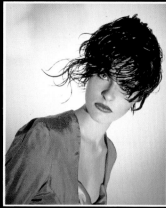

Photo: Mike Owen

above **Wild, wispy layers are gelled and left to dry naturally. By John Oliver for Schwarzkopf.**

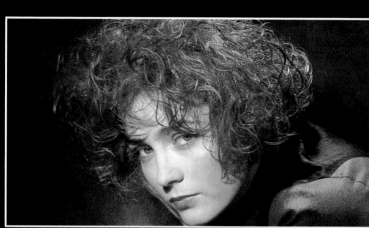

right **Copper and russet lights give warmth and glow to this layered bob. By Gary Hooker at Saks for Clynol Hair.**

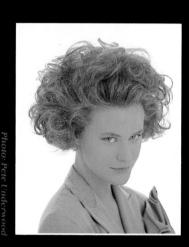

left **A soft perm gives volume and a wavy, but not tight curl. By Jeni for Clynol Hair.**

Photo: Pete Underwood

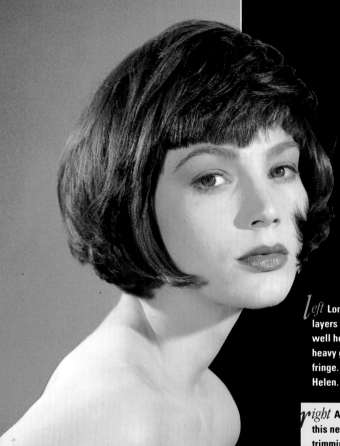

left **Long straight layers contrast well here with a heavy graduated fringe. By Ellis Helen.**

right **A bob like this needs trimming at least every six weeks to keep split ends at bay. By Caron Banfield for Wella.**

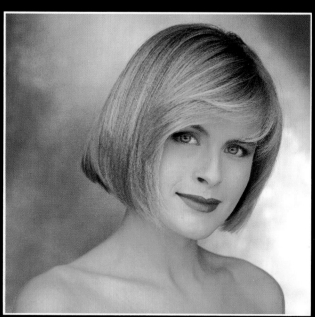

Photo: Al McDonald

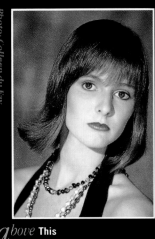

Photo: Colleen du Fay

right **Golden semi-permanent colour adds interest to chunky layers.**

above **This longer length bob with chipped-in fringe has a definite 50s feel. By Level.**

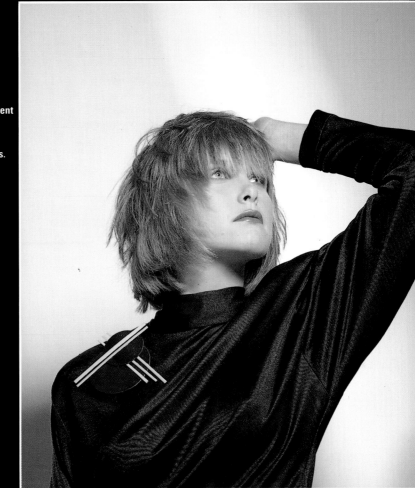

Photo: courtesy of Harmony

55

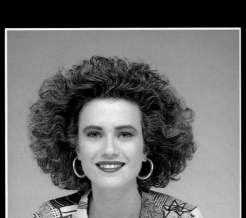

Photo: Mac

left **Ideal for curly hair, this crescent shape is based on a long page-boy style. By Karen Banfield for Clynol Hair.**

right **A dramatic forward brushed design for thick, strong hair. By Paul Mitchell.**

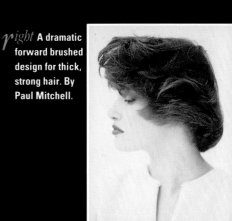

Photo: Brian Quinn

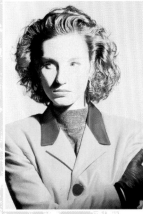

Photo: Liz McAuley

right The hair was textured around the edges but not the sides to create a sense of volume and freedom of movement. By Taylor Ferguson for Schwarzkopf.

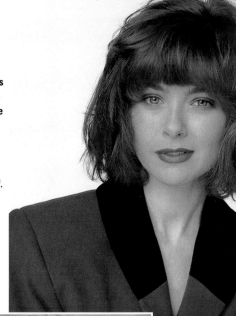

left A body perm gives the lift this style needs. By Dottie Monaghan for Clynol Hair.

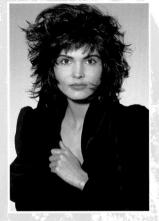

left This look is achieved by gently back-combing the crown to create height. By John Frieda.

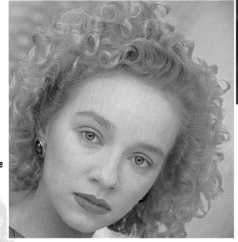

left Burnished copper curls are separated and defined using styling wax. By Sam Kelly for Schwarzkopf.

56

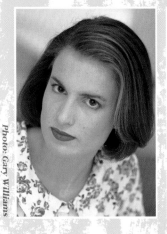

Photo: Gary Williams

left Interest has been given to brown hair by adding subtle highlights around the hairline. By Martin Gold for Wella.

right Support waves created using an acid perm. By Alison Chesterton for Zotos.

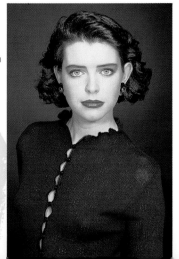

Photo: Graham Cooper

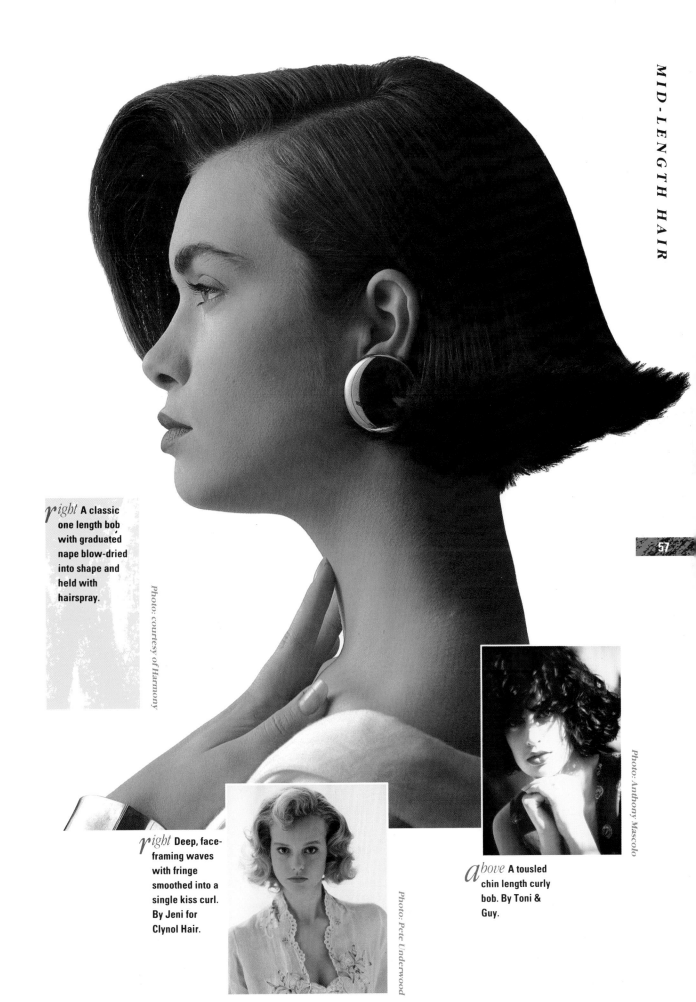

57

right **A classic one length bob with graduated nape blow-dried into shape and held with hairspray.**

Photo: courtesy of Harmony

right **Deep, face-framing waves with fringe smoothed into a single kiss curl. By Jeni for Clynol Hair.**

Photo: Pete Underwood

above **A tousled chin length curly bob. By Toni & Guy.**

Photo: Anthony Mascolo

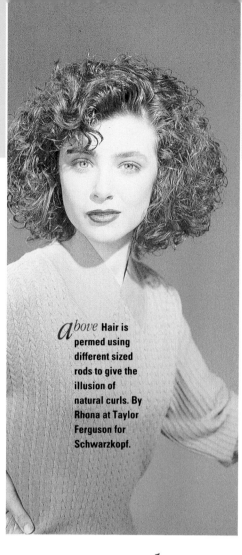

above Hair is permed using different sized rods to give the illusion of natural curls. By Rhona at Taylor Ferguson for Schwarzkopf.

right A lightly layered bob is highlighted with golden blonde. By Level.

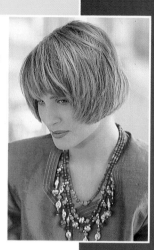

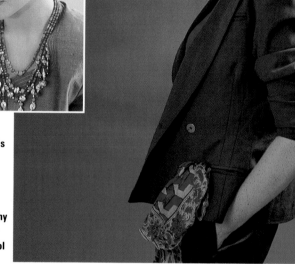

right This hair is coloured chestnut then blow-dried forwards. By Steven McCarthy of Philip's Hair Studio for Clynol Hair.

below Lots of soft curls create this pretty texture. By Philip's Hair Studio.

right This bob is dressed forwards using curling tongs.

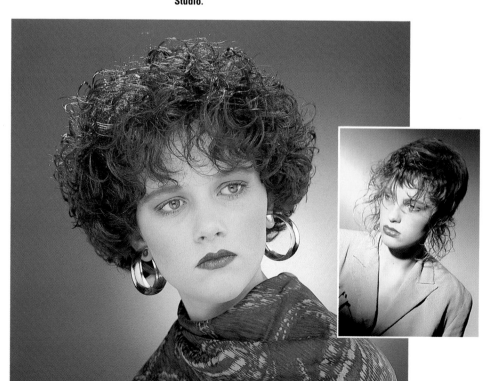

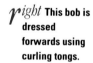

left A shaggy, carefree cut. By Rita Rusk International.

Photo: Salvadore

right Straight hair is scrunched for a wild look. By Christopher Dove at Sophisticut.

Hair is blow-dried back using a forming spray. By Richard Dalton at Claridges for Clairol.

Photo: Jeremy Enness

Photo: courtesy of BaByliss

59

left These gentle curls have been achieved with a light perm. By Jeni for Clynol Hair.

Photo: Liz McAuley

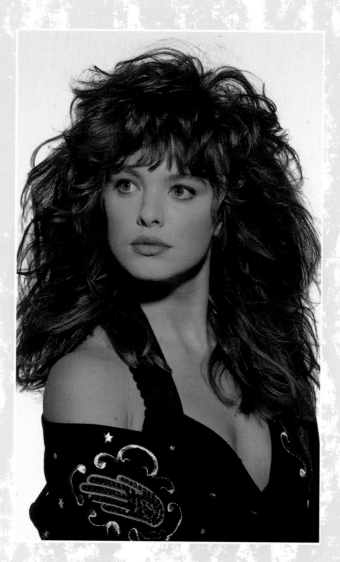

Fine, straight
hair can be
transformed into
this style by
lifting at the
roots when
drying and then
back-combing.
By John Frieda.

Long and loose styles

Historically a person's rank or social status could be deduced by the length of their hair. Long hair was for warriors, nobles and gods whilst, probably for hygiene reasons, short hair was worn by slaves and servants. Since time immemorial folklore has decreed that hair has magical properties. Caesar, when he learned of the massacre of his legionaries, swore that he would not cut his hair until their deaths had been avenged. Samson's strength was lost when Delilah cut his hair as he slept and his desire to fight was changed into servility. Over the centuries locks of hair were sacrificed to the gods in order to ward off evil spirits and demons. On a more romantic theme it was also believed that if you possessed a lock of your loved one's hair you could put him or her under your spell.

Whether women have worn their hair straight or curly has normally been a reflection of the political climate. In times of war, austere simple styles prevailed, whilst in times of plenty, extravagant curls abounded.

Hair grows at the rate of approximately half-an-inch (1 cm) a month, so very long hair is several years old. It has borne the stress of brushing, shampooing and detangling over all that time. Long hair is fragile and needs intensive conditioning and caring. The length should be trimmed regularly and the hair brushed each day using a pure, bristle brush. The bristles literally polish the hair gently spreading the natural oils from roots to ends. Combs should be wide toothed, smooth ended and of a high quality.

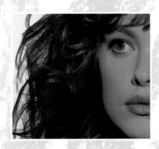

To keep hair in optimum condition you should never brush it when wet and if possible allow hair to dry naturally. Special care should be taken in the sun to protect the hair. Wear a sun hat or scarf or use a cream or gel with a built-in sunscreen.

Whilst hot irons and other electrical styling equipment are perfect for creating extravagant curly looks, their use should be restricted to perhaps once or twice a week, and they should not be used on a daily basis or the hair could be damaged. Remember if your hair is naturally curly, growing it longer will increase its weight and this will tend to straighten the curl. So if you want to maximize your curls choose a layered cut. Also avoid over-zealous brushing of curly hair, as this will tend to straighten the curl and sometimes turn it to frizz. Instead choose an 'Afro' wide-toothed comb which should be gently raked through, thus preserving the movement. If the hair is fine and thin, the best long cut has feathered layers which help to give an appearance of added volume and texture.

Here you will find a stunning selection of cascading curls, shimmering, swinging styles to inspire you to grow your hair long.

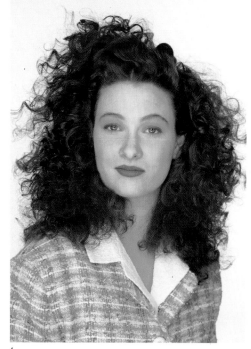

*a*bove **A perm creates a mass of tumbling curls. By John Richardson of John Oliver for Schwarzkopf.**

*b*elow **This wonderful mane of golden curls is achieved by perming using bendy rods. By Lisa Waite at Del Capello for Wella.**

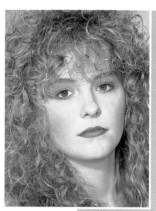

Photo: Mike Davis

*r*ight **Pre-Raphaelite waves dressed over to one side. By Philip's Hair Studio.**

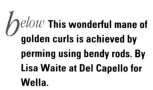

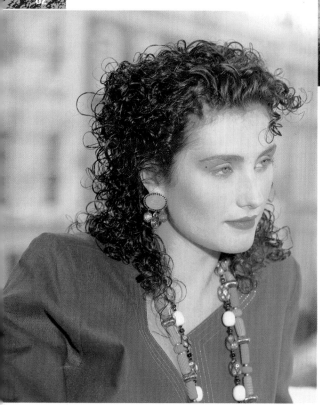

Photo: Arthur Moulding

*l*eft **Defined waves were permed by using reverse spiral winding on to chopsticks. By Stephen Wake at Level for Schwarzkopf.**

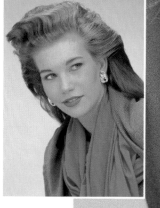

*l*eft **A flexible styling brush and blow-drying achieves this smooth look. By Keith Harris for Clairol Professional.**

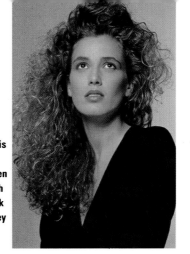

right This look is defined by first blow-drying then separating each curl with a slick of wax. By Carey Temple McAdam.

below A perm creates cascades of voluminous waves. By Billy Shear at Ocean Boulevard.

left The top is back-combed and length allowed to fall free. By Taylor Ferguson.

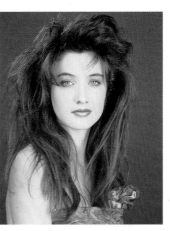

right Long, straight hair needn't be just that! With a little back-combing at the roots you can create this soft, sultry style. By Mark Lorrell at Fields.

Photo: Raphael

Photo: Bill Savoy

63

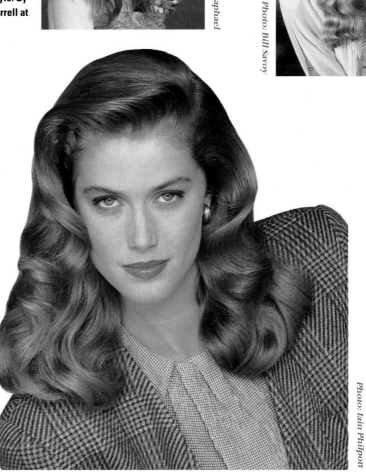

right Intensive conditioning at least once a week is vital to keep this style in optimum condition. By Karen Banfield for Wella.

Photo: Iain Philpott

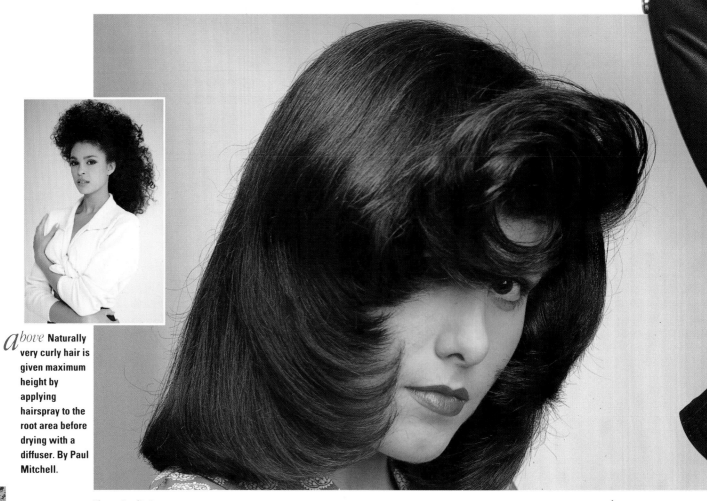

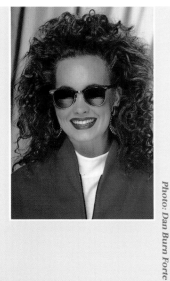

*a*bove Naturally very curly hair is given maximum height by applying hairspray to the root area before drying with a diffuser. By Paul Mitchell.

Photo: Leslie Lowery

*b*elow more controlled curl is achieved by separating each section with styling wax. By Fields.

*r*ight This shoulder-length hair is spiral permed for a spectacular result. By Melvyn & Friends.

*b*elow Soft, springy curls are created by an 'air' perm which uses a protein spray and the oxygen in the air as a neutralizer. By Mark Lovell at Fields.

*a*bove This luxuriant glossy sheen is achieved by using a warm mahogany semi-permanent conditioning colourant. By Angela Miller at Y Salon for Wella.

Photo: Dan Burn Forte

Photo: David Darling

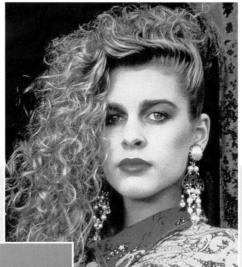

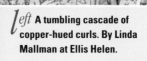

*l*eft A tumbling cascade of copper-hued curls. By Linda Mallman at Ellis Helen.

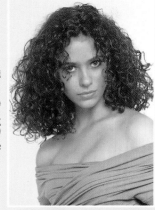

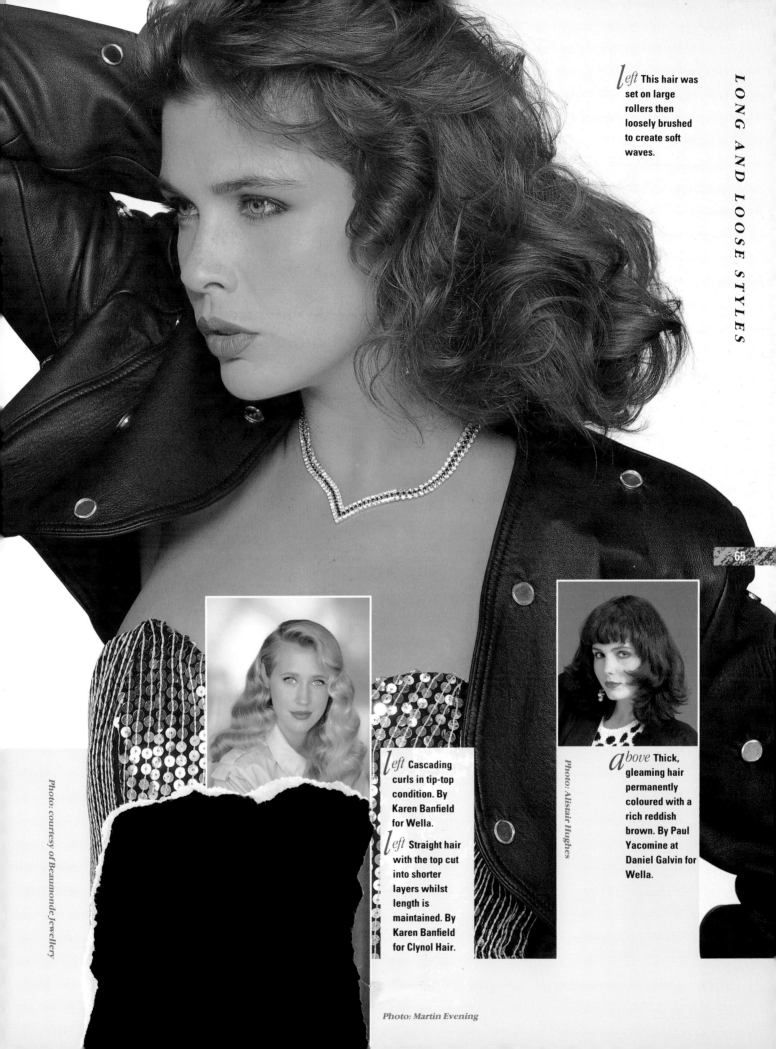

left **This hair was set on large rollers then loosely brushed to create soft waves.**

65

Photo: courtesy of Beaumonde Jewellery

left **Cascading curls in tip-top condition. By Karen Banfield for Wella.**

left **Straight hair with the top cut into shorter layers whilst length is maintained. By Karen Banfield for Clynol Hair.**

Photo: Alistair Hughes

above **Thick, gleaming hair permanently coloured with a rich reddish brown. By Paul Yacomine at Daniel Galvin for Wella.**

Photo: Martin Evening

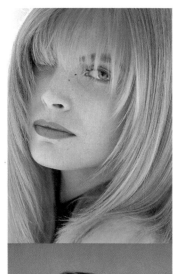

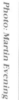

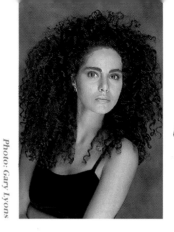

Photo: Gary Lyons

left Naturally very curly hair is spiral tonged for additional bounce. By Jeanne Braa for Paul Mitchell.

right Two sleek and straight face-framing styles. Above: by Edmonds Below: by Stephen Wake at Level. Both for Schwarzkopf.

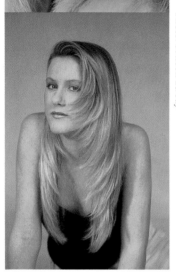

Photo: Colleen du Fay

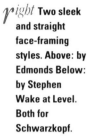

66

Photo: Martin Evening

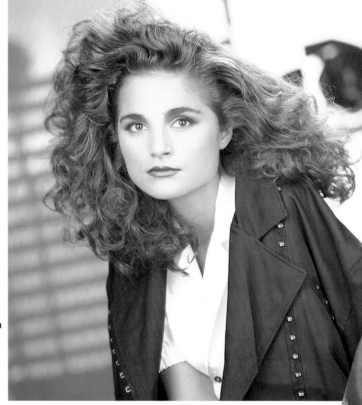

right Colour enhanced with a permanent mahogany shade. By Karen Banfield for Clynol Hair.

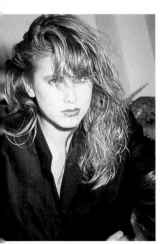

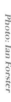

left Straight layered hair dried by applying mousse and scrunching. By Carey Temple McAdam.

Photo: Ian Forster

Photo: Martin Evening

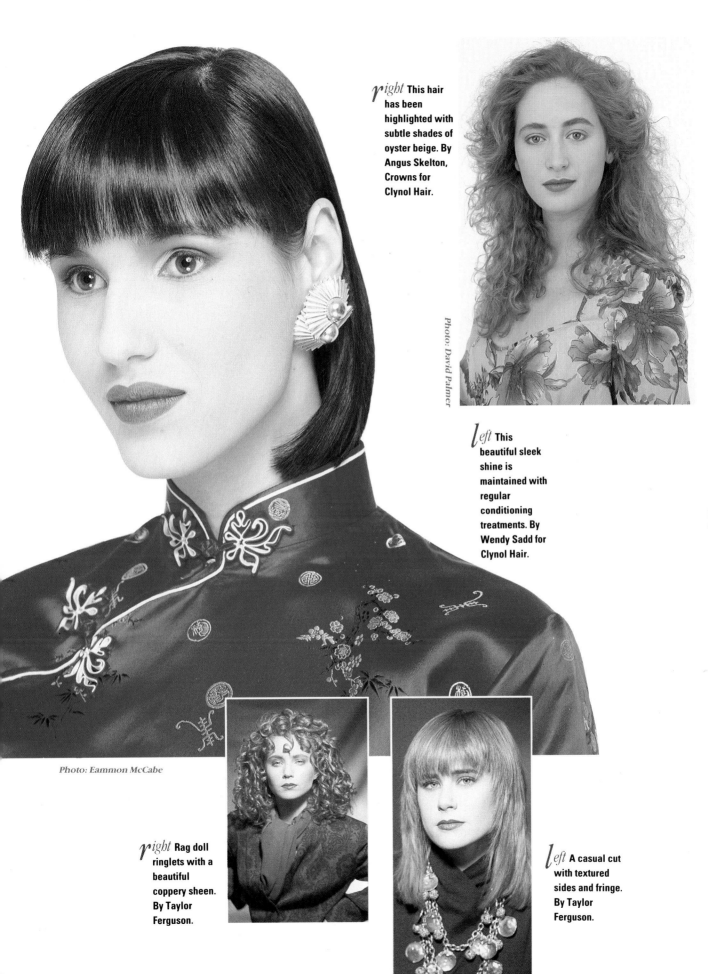

right This hair has been highlighted with subtle shades of oyster beige. By Angus Skelton, Crowns for Clynol Hair.

Photo: David Palmer

left This beautiful sleek shine is maintained with regular conditioning treatments. By Wendy Sadd for Clynol Hair.

Photo: Eammon McCabe

right Rag doll ringlets with a beautiful coppery sheen. By Taylor Ferguson.

left A casual cut with textured sides and fringe. By Taylor Ferguson.

67

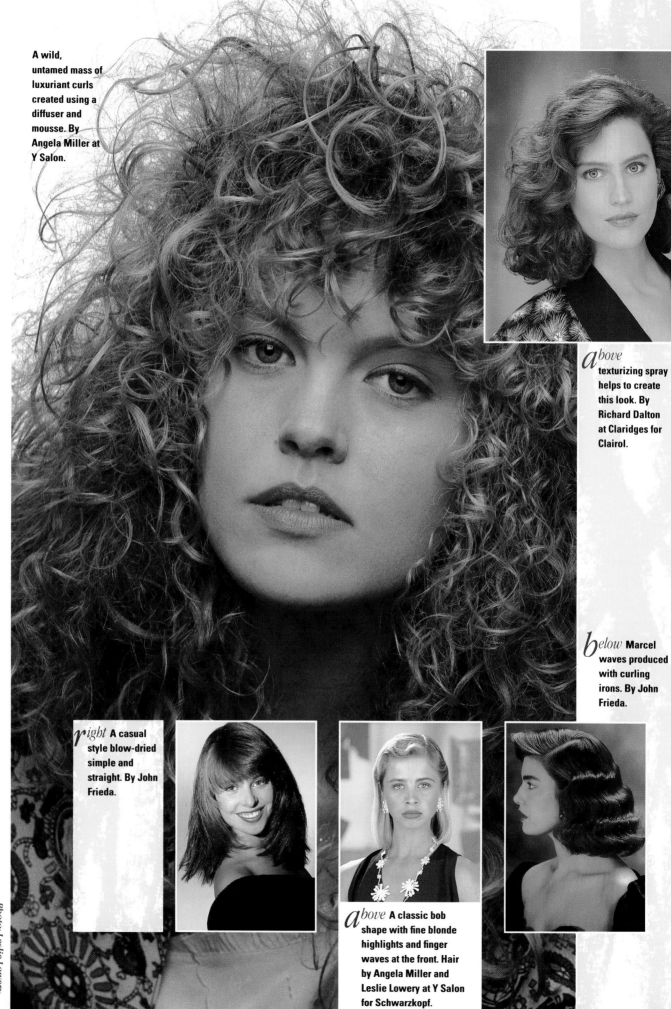

A wild, untamed mass of luxuriant curls created using a diffuser and mousse. By Angela Miller at Y Salon.

68

*a*bove texturizing spray helps to create this look. By Richard Dalton at Claridges for Clairol.

*b*elow Marcel waves produced with curling irons. By John Frieda.

*r*ight A casual style blow-dried simple and straight. By John Frieda.

*a*bove A classic bob shape with fine blonde highlights and finger waves at the front. Hair by Angela Miller and Leslie Lowery at Y Salon for Schwarzkopf.

Photo: Leslie Lowery

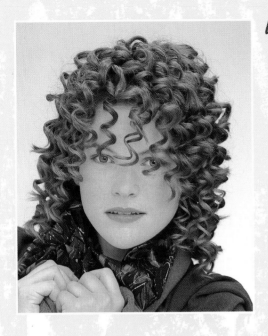

left **Bendy rollers produce this rag-doll type curl. By Keith Harris for Clairol Professional.**

right **A shaggy, controlled look dried back from the forehead. By Carey Temple McAdam.**

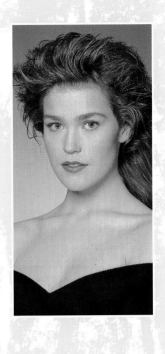

right **This hair was conditioned both before and after perming to achieve a strong, defined curl. By Graham Webb International for Clynol Hair.**

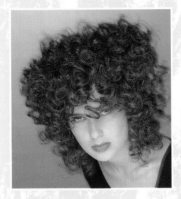

below **A mass of curly locks was created by setting the hair on smallish rollers and brushing through very lightly.**

Photo: Gary Lyons

below **Slim curling tongs and a little expertise made these flowing curls.**

69

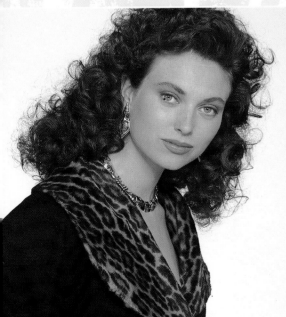

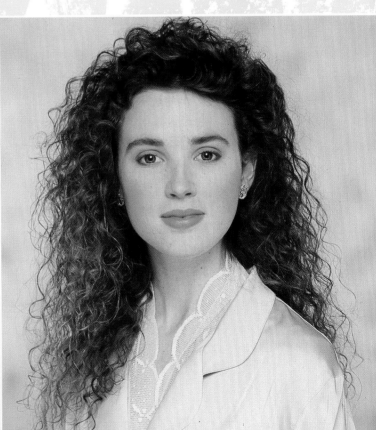

Photo: courtesy of Vendome Jewellery

Photo: courtesy BaByliss Professional

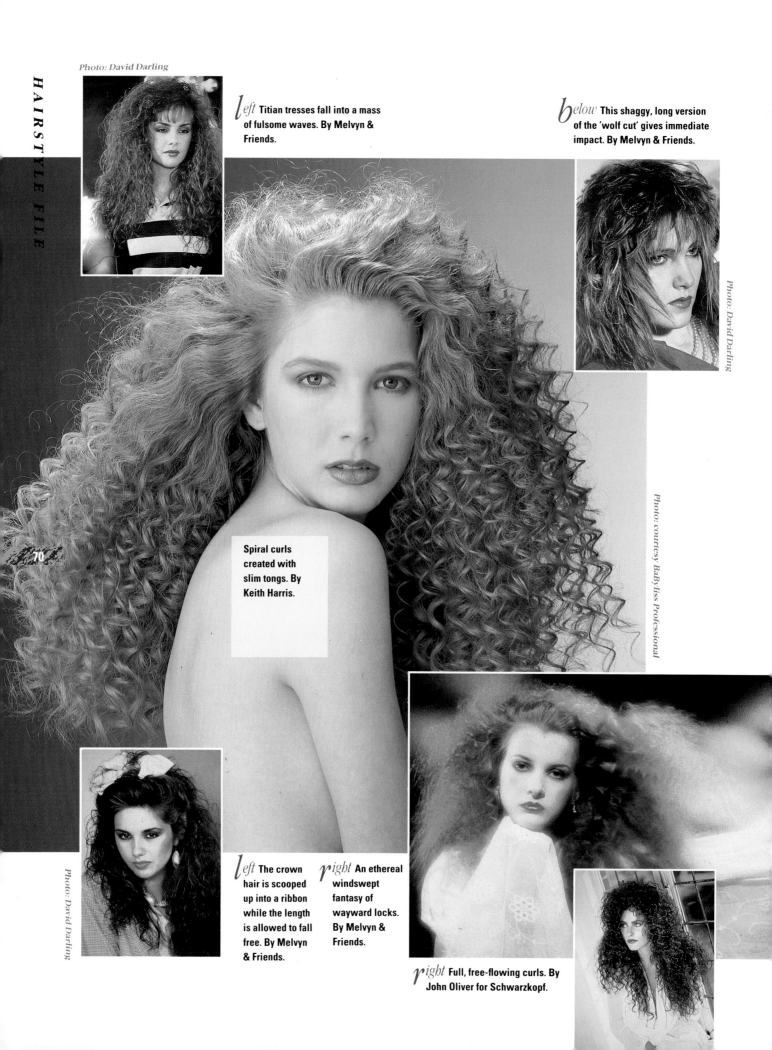

Photo: David Darling

left Titian tresses fall into a mass of fulsome waves. By Melvyn & Friends.

below This shaggy, long version of the 'wolf cut' gives immediate impact. By Melvyn & Friends.

Photo: David Darling

Photo: courtesy BaByliss Professional

70

Spiral curls created with slim tongs. By Keith Harris.

Photo: David Darling

left The crown hair is scooped up into a ribbon while the length is allowed to fall free. By Melvyn & Friends.

right An ethereal windswept fantasy of wayward locks. By Melvyn & Friends.

right Full, free-flowing curls. By John Oliver for Schwarzkopf.

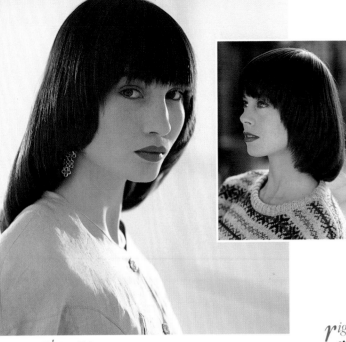

left This beautifully conditioned hair lays sleek and shimmering. By Lewis Jubenville for Wella.

Photo: Al Macdonald

above This graduated long line bob is blow-dried using a texturizing spray. By Richard Dalton at Claridges for Clairol Professional.

right Chic and stunning, perfect condition is vital for this style. By Mark Jones at Ellis Helen.

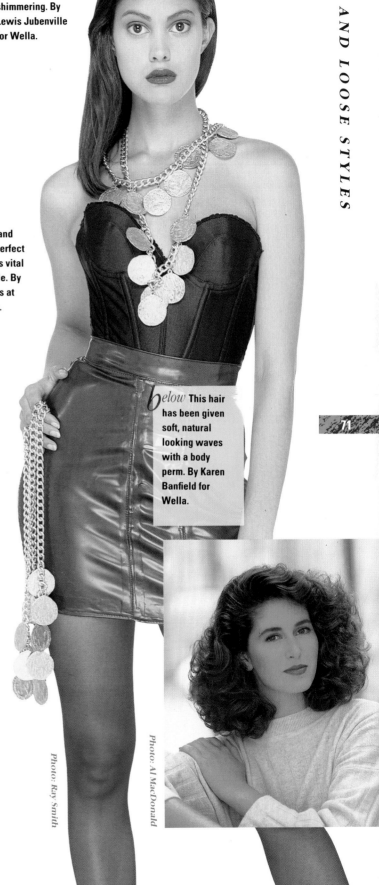

below This hair has been given soft, natural looking waves with a body perm. By Karen Banfield for Wella.

below A slightly wild and tousled look on permed, highlighted hair. By Melvyn & Friends.

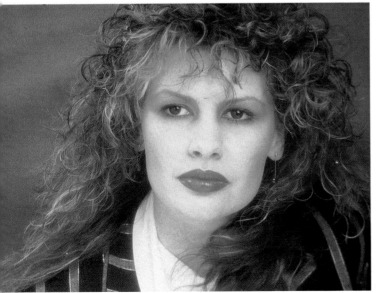

Photo: David Darling

Photo: Ray Smith

Photo: Al MacDonald

73

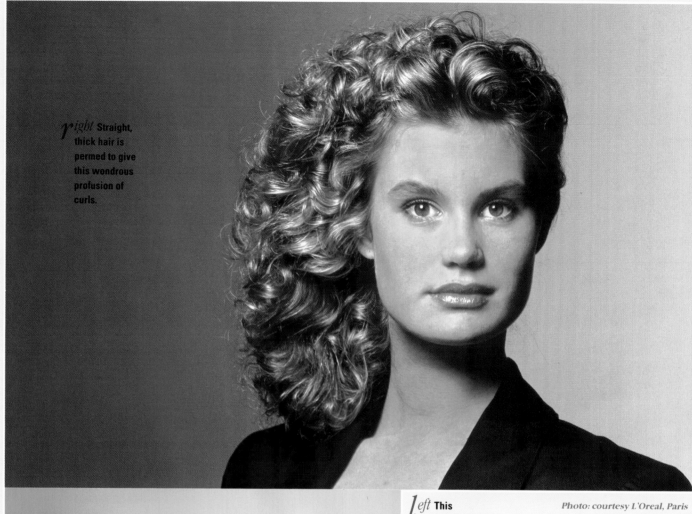

right Straight, thick hair is permed to give this wondrous profusion of curls.

Photo: courtesy L'Oreal, Paris

left **This beautiful natural shade of blonde is achieved by lightening. By Rebecca Cazaly for Wella.**

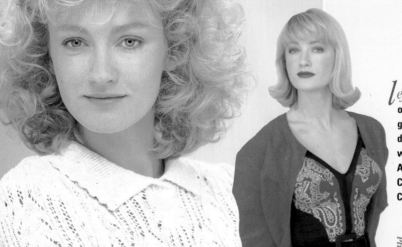

left **Subtle lights of gold and sand give a feeling of depth and warmth. By Angus Skelton at Crowns for Clynol Hair.**

Photo: Alistair Hughes

Photo: David Palmer

*b*elow **An abundance of ruffled ringlets. By Toni & Guy.**

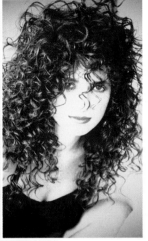

Photo: Anthony Mascolo

Photo: Brian Quinn

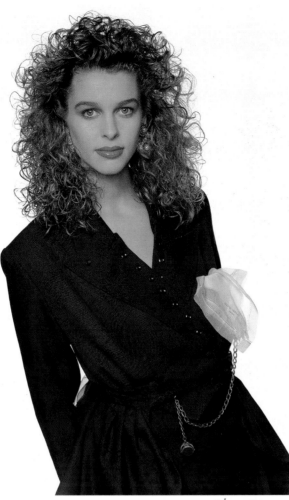

Photo: Anthony Mascolo

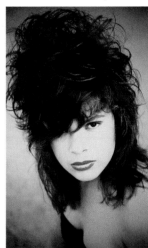

*a*bove **This style has plenty of volume on top with length left a little straighter. By Toni & Guy.**

73

*a*bove **This permed hair was twisted at the roots and dried with a diffuser. By Taylor Ferguson for Schwarzkopf.**

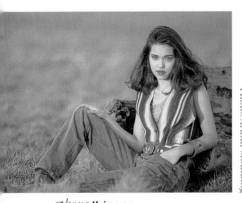

Photo: Arthur Moulding

*a*bove **Hairspray is applied to the roots and then the hair is blow-dried with the head tipped forward. By Lisa Johansen at Macmillan.**

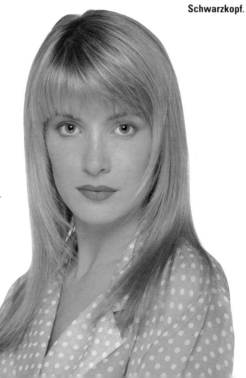

*r*ight **This silky, fine, straight hair is fringed and feathered for extra body before being allowed to dry naturally.**

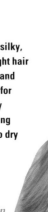

Photo: courtesy of Silvikrin

Photo: Arthur Moulding

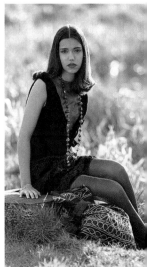

*r*ight **For a sleek look, dry hair using a vent brush to bend the ends out a little. By Lisa Johansen at Macmillan.**

below **Naturally wavy locks left to fall free and loose. By Ellis Helen.**

right **Casual blonde lights give this long bob a soft, shimmering look. By Paul Edmonds for Schwarzkopf.**

Photo: Peter Pfänder

below **A perm creates beautiful waves on perfectly conditioned hair. By Helen Blackburn at Ellis Helen for Wella.**

74

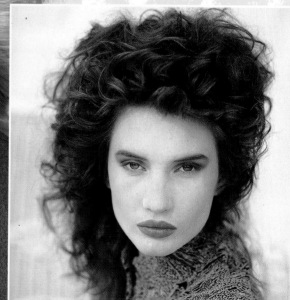

Photo: Gary Williams

*r*ight **These deep, sensuous waves fall soft and loose. By Jeanne Braa at Paul Mitchell.**

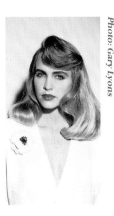

Photo: Gary Lyons

*l*eft **Heavy layers are left throughout the crown and ends thinned for a wispy look. By Gary Hooker at Saks for Clynol Hair.**

Photo: Melissa Halstead

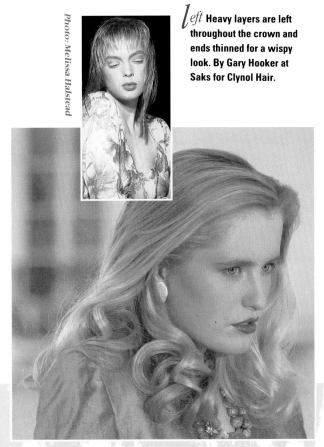

Photo: Colleen du Fay

*a*bove **Hair is blow-dried under for this smooth, silky look. By Level.**

75

*b*elow **Highlighted hair is given exotic waves and volume by perming. By Patrick Cameron at Alan Paul for Wella.**

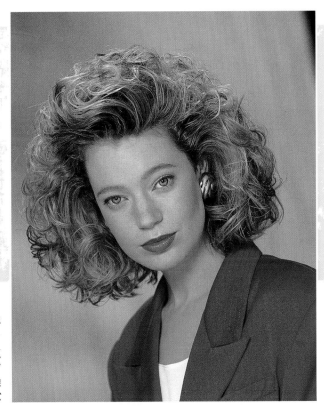

Photo: Adrian Fiebig

*l*eft **Brown hair is given a warm russet glow and rich glossy sheen using a conditioning colourant. By Anna Longaretti for Wella.**

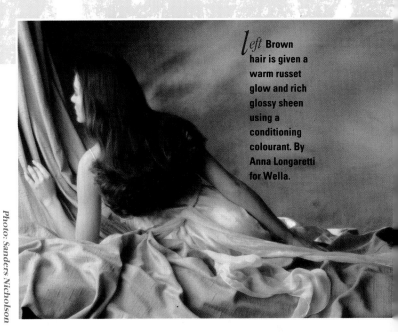

Photo: Sanders Nicholson

*l*eft **A perm can turn a head of straight hair into an amazing mass of bouncing curls. By Fields.**

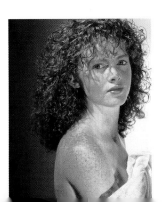

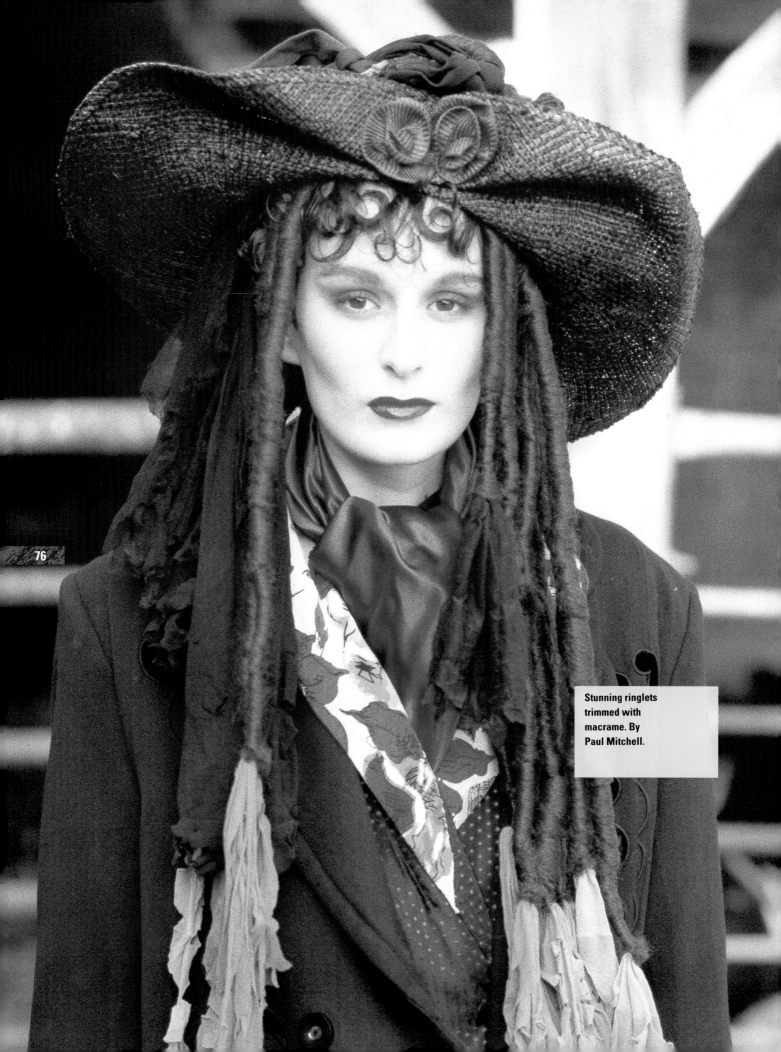

Stunning ringlets trimmed with macrame. By Paul Mitchell.

Dressed styles

Braided hair was first seen in the fourteenth century and this was usually in the form of two thick plaits

coiled around the ears. During this period high rounded foreheads were considered beautiful and young women would pluck the hair from the hair line in order to create this effect. In this era hairstyles became more complex with beribboned plaits coiled extravagantly at the back of the head. As the fashion for plucked hairlines diminished, hair was dressed in large chignons. Very often the side hair was cut short and waved to give a striking contrast to the sleekness of the back.

Towards the end of the fifteenth century curls had been replaced with hair caught tightly back from the forehead and secured over oval frames. Soft tendrils, called love-locks were left to fall in front of the ears.

By the late sixteenth century high ruff collars had became the fashion and hair was then back-combed and supported on wire cradles.

Padded rolls were also used to give volume and additional height. Elizabeth I's favourite hairstyle was a heart-shaped concoction of masses of tiny curls which was set off by a fan-shaped lace collar.

Today, the advent of numerous styling products – mousses, gels and particularly hairspray – have all helped to make the hairdressers' job easier. A style that might have taken several hours to dress in days gone by can now be created quickly and easily.

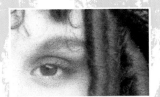

Covered bands provide one of the simplest ways to put hair up yourself and gives a good basis for further dressing. Once a ponytail is secured, a combination of twisting, coiling, curling, plaiting and looping techniques can be used to create an endless variety of looks. Combs, slides, ribbons and scarves can all be intertwined to give added interest.

When dressing hair up, it is essential that it is properly prepared or the finished result won't be glossy and sleek. To give the style the right foundation, root lift is required. This can be achieved easily at home by using a combination of styling products and heated appliances. However, some people prefer to use a traditional setting technique. To do this damp hair should be set on rollers going back away from hairline. The lower back should be set on rollers going in an upward direction. The hair is dried thoroughly and allowed to 'cool' whilst the rollers are still in place.

Overleaf you will find a selection of dressed styles to suit every occasion.

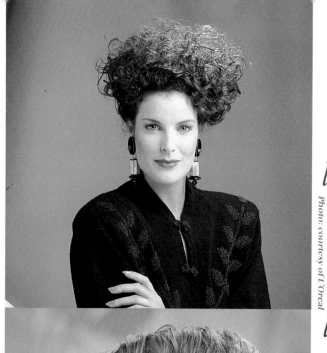

Photo: courtesy of L'Oreal

left Extravagant permed curls create this ultra-sophisticated look.

right Here the hair is swept loosely up with a small ponytail softening the line. By Ellis Helen.

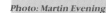

Photo: Martin Evening

left Rich exotically coloured hair is finger-dried for this picture of casual glamour. By Paul Edmonds at Edmonds for Schwarzkopf.

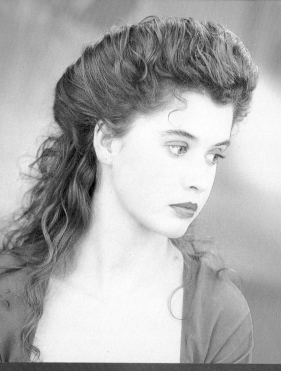

Photo: Martin Evening

right Shoulder length hair is dressed with a gentle wave movement through the front and with delicate rolls of hair on top. By Angela Miller and Leslie Lowery at Y Salon for Schwarzkopf.

below This ultra-sophisticated style incorporates a quiff, plaits and basket-weave sections. By Carey Temple McAdam.

left Rich golds and browns give definition to these curls. By Rebecca Cazaly for Wella.

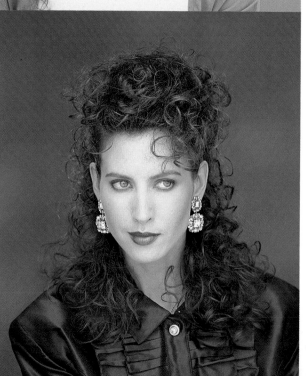

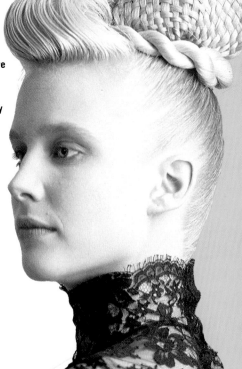

Photo: Ursula Steiger

An elegant look achieved by hair softly swept into waves in the front and a sleek roll through the back. By Steven McCarthy at Philip's Hair Studio for Clynol Hair.

Photo: Colleen du Fay

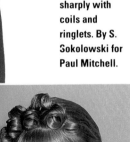

below A straight fringe contrasts sharply with coils and ringlets. By S. Sokolowski for Paul Mitchell.

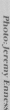

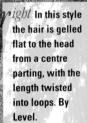

right In this style the hair is gelled flat to the head from a centre parting, with the length twisted into loops. By Level.

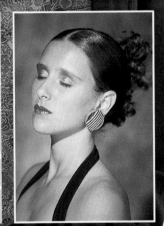

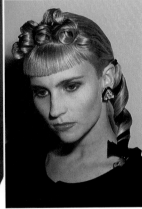

Photo: Gary Lyons

above An abundance of full, soft curls. By Steven Wake at Level.

Photo: Jeremy Enness

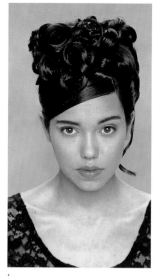

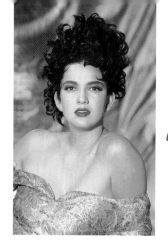

left Height is created at the top and sides with looped curls. By Beverly Kyprianou at Cobella for Schwarzkopf.

right These glossy auburn curls are piled up high and wide. By Guy Kremer at French Connection.

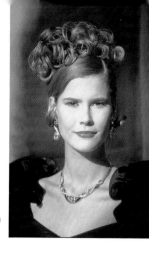

Photo: Ursula Steiger

left This blonde hair is highlighted with a sandy gold to give depth and warmth. By Angus Skelton at Crowns for Clynol Hair.

below This pretty mass of curls is coloured damson brown and gold. By Geoff Smith at 'Smiths for Hair' for Wella.

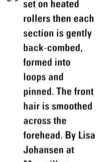

above The hair is set on heated rollers then each section is gently back-combed, formed into loops and pinned. The front hair is smoothed across the forehead. By Lisa Johansen at Macmillan.

Photo: Eammon McCabe

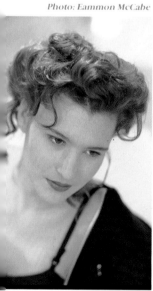

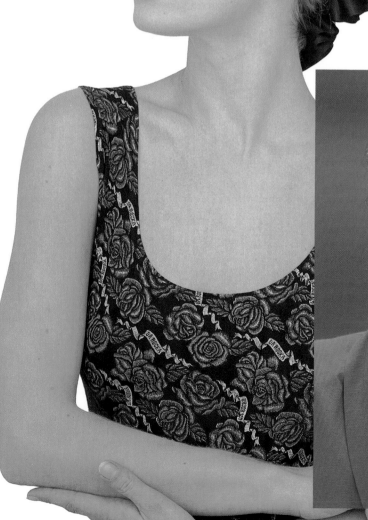

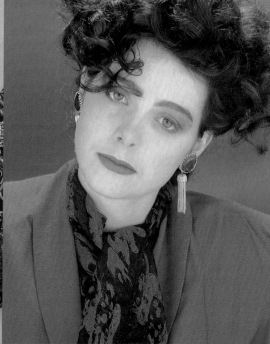

above A soft, summery style is held in place with hairspray. By Wendy Sadd for Clynol Hair.

Photo: David Palmer

Photo: Philip Ollerensh

right This hair is clasped with a ribbon and dressed into a mass of curls. By Paul Edmonds at Edmonds for Schwarzkopf.

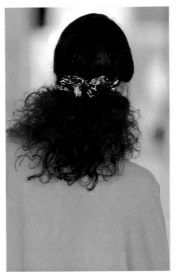

Photo: Peter Pfander

below A striking upswept style with a ruffled finish. By Fields.

below This style is finger-waved at the front and back-combed at the crown. By Angela Miller at Y Salon.

81

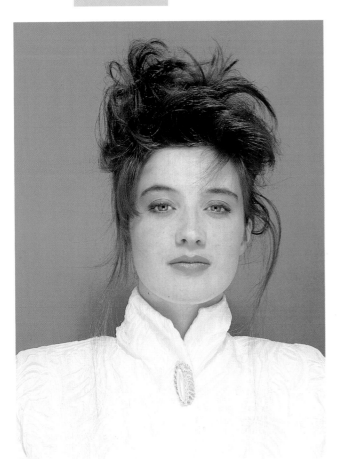

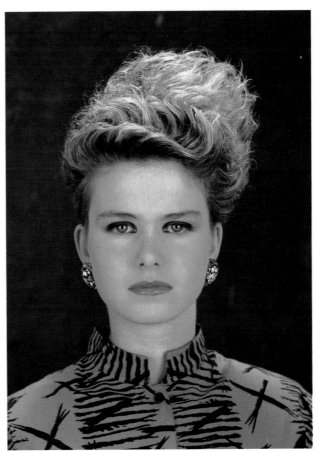

Photo: Leslie Lowery

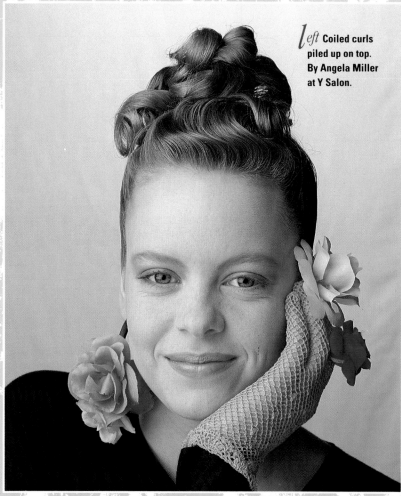

left Coiled curls piled up on top. By Angela Miller at Y Salon.

Photo: Leslie Lowery

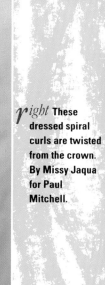

right These dressed spiral curls are twisted from the crown. By Missy Jaqua for Paul Mitchell.

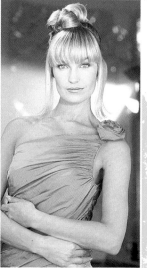

Photo: Martin Evening

above A nordic blonde with looped curls. By Terry Calvert at Clipso for Schwarzkopf.

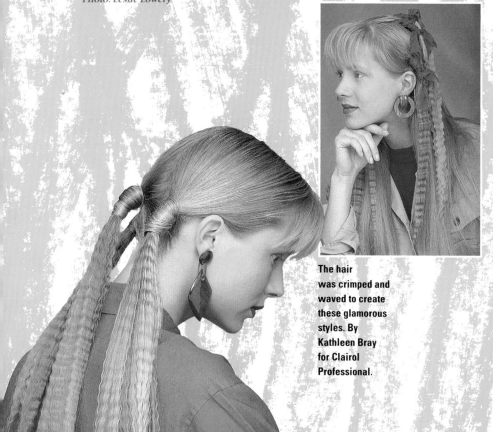

The hair was crimped and waved to create these glamorous styles. By Kathleen Bray for Clairol Professional.

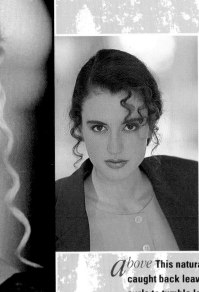

right Here the crown hair is dressed then crimped, and the lower hair crimped and left to fall loosely. By Kathleen Bray for Clairol Professional.

Photo: Peter Pfander

above This naturally wavy hair is caught back leaving random curls to tumble loosely. By Paul Edmonds at Edmonds for Schwarzkopf.

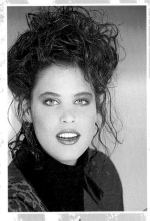

above This long hair is casually scooped up. By Level.

left A wild look created with back-brushing. By Carey Temple McAdam.

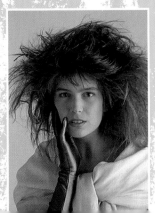

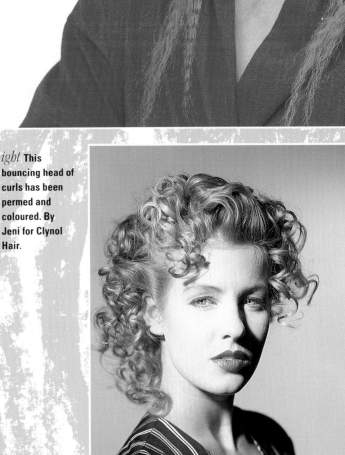

83

right This bouncing head of curls has been permed and coloured. By Jeni for Clynol Hair.

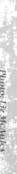

Photo: Liz McAuley

right These
layered curls are
finished with
styling wax. By
Christopher Dove
at Sophisticut.

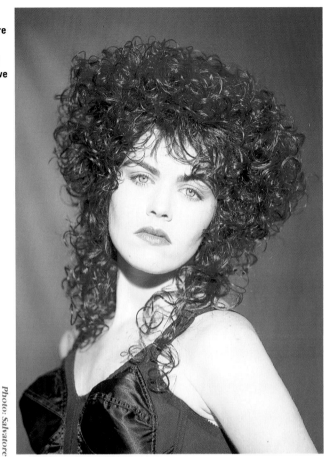

Photo: Salvatore

above Natural
tresses tumble
from a soft
French pleat. By
Angela Miller at
Y Salon.

below This hair
is permed then
scrunch-dried
for a pretty look.
By Fields.

84

right A shock of
tiny tendrils
cascade around
the face and
neck. By Rita
Rusk
International.

below A small
section of hair is
twisted and used
to 'catch' hair at
the nape. By
Denice Hansen
for Paul
Mitchell.

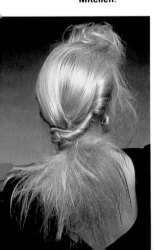

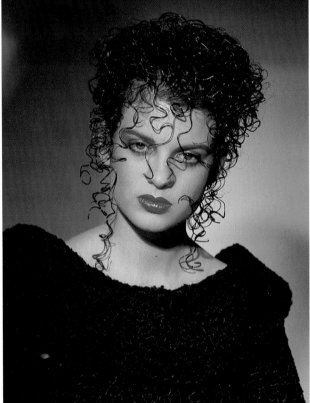

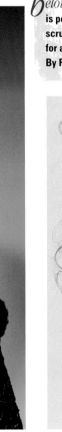

Photo: Jack Cutter

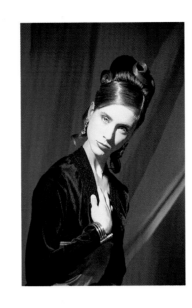

left A sleek front with curls on top creates this eye-catching look. By Guy Kremer at French Connection.

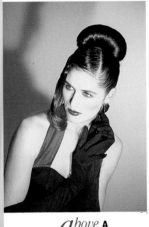

Photo: Leslie Lowery

above A sophisticated, elegant rolled bun with the length left down. By Guy Kremer at French Connection.

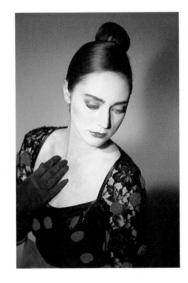

left The classic silky, shiny top knot. By Guy Kremer at French Connection.

85

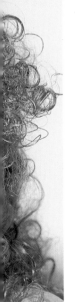

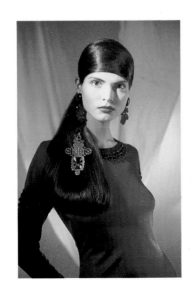

left Glossy hair is wrapped round the crown with the length left to fall over one shoulder. By John Richardson for Schwarzkopf.

below For this elegant evening look the hair is swept back and twisted to form a 'knot' chignon. By Paul Edmonds at Edmonds for Schwarzkopf.

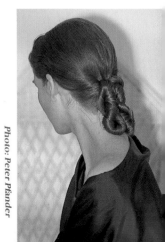

Photo: Peter Pfänder

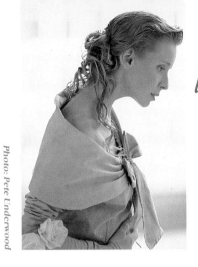

Photo: Pete Underwood

left **The crown hair is moulded into shape and the length fastened into loose tendrils at the nape. By Jeni for Clynol Hair.**

right **The hair is drawn tightly into a low ponytail. The length is then tonged and curls loosely released. By John Oliver for Schwarzkopf.**

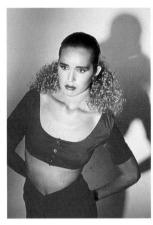

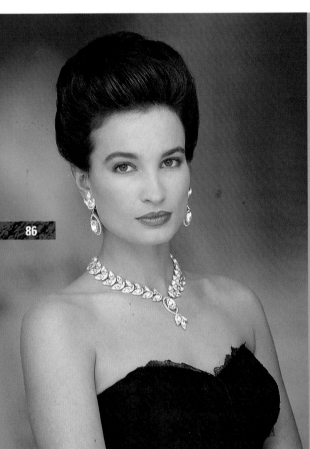

86

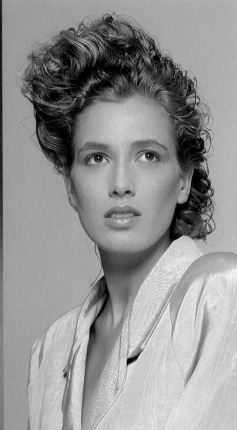

left **Naturally curly locks are finger-waved at the front and caught up with combs. By Carey Temple McAdam.**

above **This back-combed upswept look is held in place with hairspray. By Richard Dalton at Claridges for Clairol.**

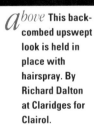

right **Glamorous bouffant waves cascade softly in this style. By John Oliver for Schwarzkopf.**

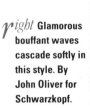

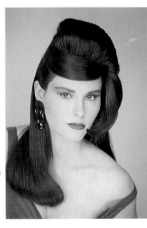

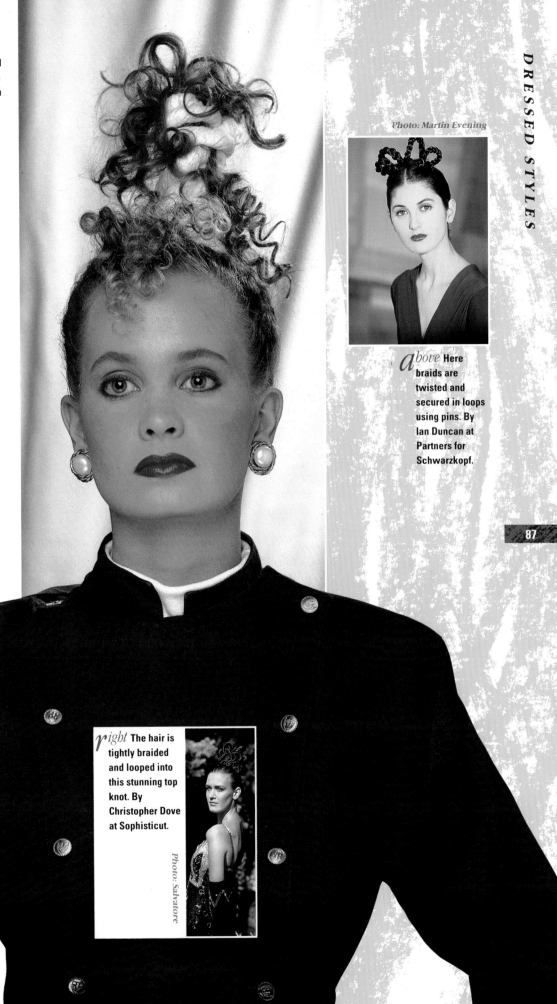

right **Beautiful upswept curls are laced with ribbons. By Fields.**

Photo: Martin Evening

above **The hair is pin set over cotton wool using mousse and the loops of the twisted spiral curls intertwined and woven into each other. By Ian Duncan at Partners for Schwarzkopf.**

Photo: Martin Evening

above **Here braids are twisted and secured in loops using pins. By Ian Duncan at Partners for Schwarzkopf.**

87

right **The hair is tightly braided and looped into this stunning top knot. By Christopher Dove at Sophisticut.**

Photo: Salvatore

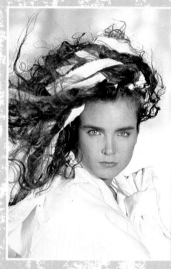

above **Romantic curls are woven with white ribbons. By Carey Temple McAdam.**

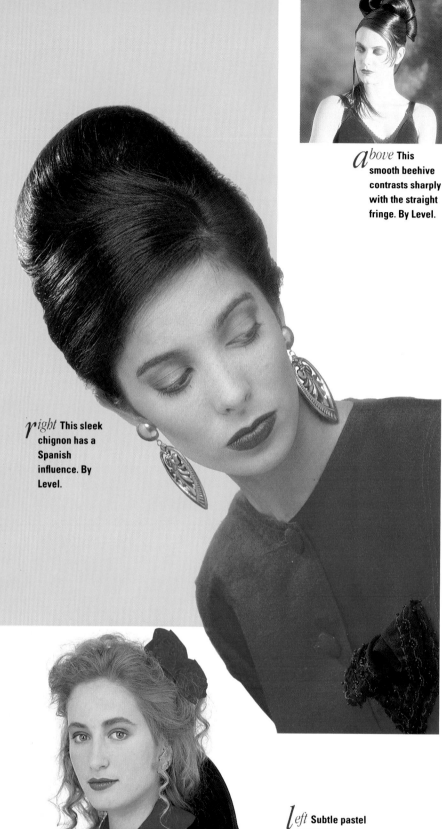

right **This sleek chignon has a Spanish influence. By Level.**

above **This smooth beehive contrasts sharply with the straight fringe. By Level.**

above **Side pieces are left free to soften this upswept look. By Andrew Collinge.**

Photo: David Palmer

left **Subtle pastel highlights enhance this mass of carefree curls. By Angus Skelton of Crowns for Clynol Hair.**

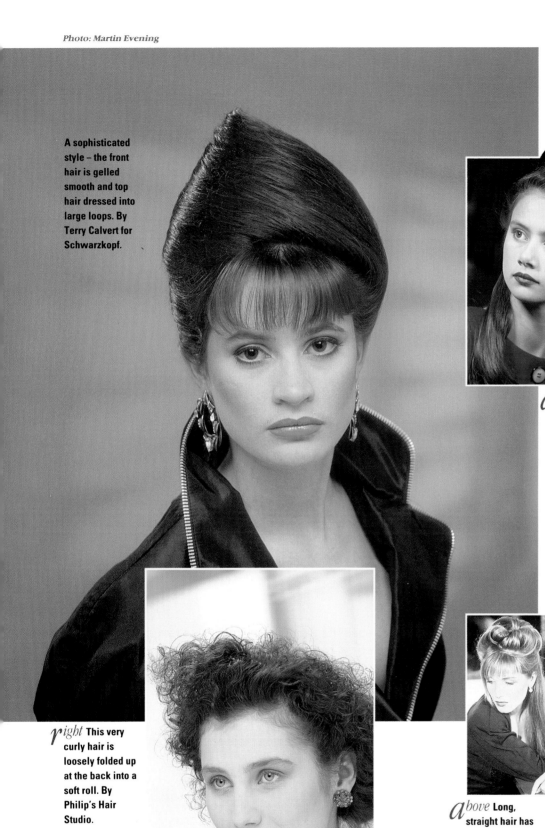

A sophisticated style – the front hair is gelled smooth and top hair dressed into large loops. By Terry Calvert for Schwarzkopf.

below A blonde bob is transformed by a mass of large curls. By Guy Kremer for Schwarzkopf.

above A simple top knot dresses up very long locks for a lovely evening creation. By Guy Kremer at French Connection.

89

right This very curly hair is loosely folded up at the back into a soft roll. By Philip's Hair Studio.

above Long, straight hair has been graduated through its length, then the top sections pinned into large coils and loops. By Alison White at Dom Migele.

Photo: Rosalind Gaunt

Photo: Martin Evening

above The hair is delicately caught from the sides, twisted and coiled like embroidery before lacing with braid. By Paul Edmonds at Edmonds for Schwarzkopf.

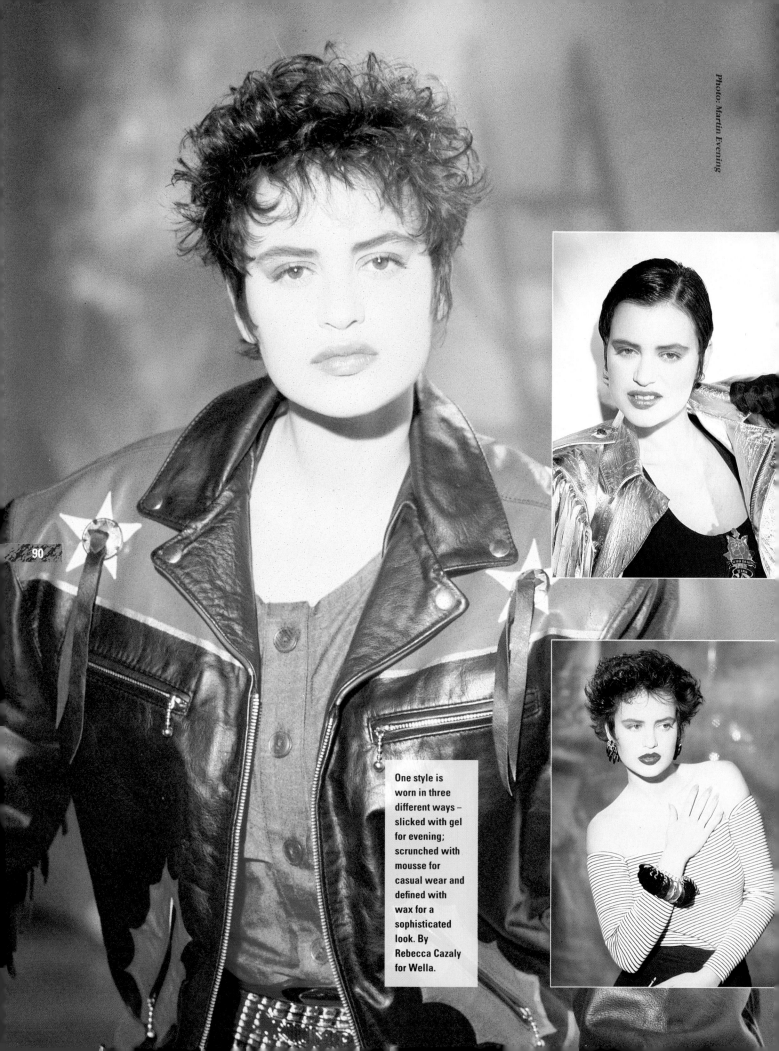

Photo: Martin Evening

90

One style is worn in three different ways – slicked with gel for evening; scrunched with mousse for casual wear and defined with wax for a sophisticated look. By Rebecca Cazaly for Wella.

Transformations

Choosing a hair cut that will adapt so that it can be worn in several ways is essential in this day and age. It's ideal if your hair can be transformed quickly and easily to suit your mood and the occasion. Expert cuts that are easy-to-convert enable you to create dramatic changes with the flick of a comb, the use of hair appliances and styling products.

Whatever cut you choose – short, mid-length or long – you should be able to style it in a variety of ways. Try blow-drying in totally different directions: away from the face, over to the side, or forward. Change the parting from left to right or centre for immediate impact. Get lift and volume from the root area by drying against the growth direction and finger-style for a less tailored look.

If your hair is naturally curly with a frizzy texture, apply mousse/gel to towel-dried hair to make it easier to style. Remember curls should always be dried with a diffuser as a normal dryer will just make the hair even frizzier. A wide-toothed comb is essential too – a normal comb will mean more frizz.

Permed hair should only be shampooed every three days or so, more often will dry it out. To re-activate curls between washing, mist hair with water spray and scrunch or loosely tie up, letting tendrils fall freely around your face.

If you want to ring the changes on your colour without a commitment try a 'convertible' cut with colour. Pioneered by Vidal Sassoon, this technique tones subtle shades of colour together so the look can be totally different depending on the way you choose to style your hair. It is based on the principle of the tide – brushing your hair one way reveals one shade, brush it another way and the hues are slightly different. Convertible colour is the ideal way to introduce yourself to change because the colour can be as delicate as you like and applied in different ways.

Mid-to-long hair is perhaps the easiest to transform. Bend your head forward and brush the hair up to the crown. Secure it in a covered band or 'scrunchie'. To soften the look, release small sections of hair and allow to fall free. Plaits are another easy way to change your style. A simple plait is done by dividing hair into three sections and crossing in sequence. A weave plait is more complicated as new sections are introduced from the side of head into each new weave. Get a friend to help and you will soon become proficient at this technique.

An easy way to dress hair differently is by using bands, bows and ribbons and the best hunting ground for accessories is large department stores. Look in the jewellery, haircare and haberdashery departments for unusual bits and bobs.

Here we show how you can make a dramatic change by selecting a new way of styling. Scrunching, blow-drying, straightening, curling – just see how easy it is to make a style look different . . . .

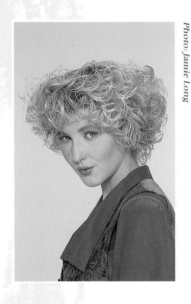

Photo: Jamie Long

left **Playful curls are shaped flat to the top of the head.**

right **Hair is slicked back to the nape and the fringe curled. By Stephen Wake for Schwarzkopf.**

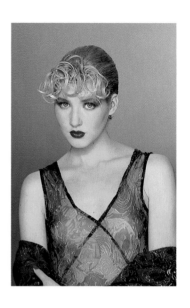

92

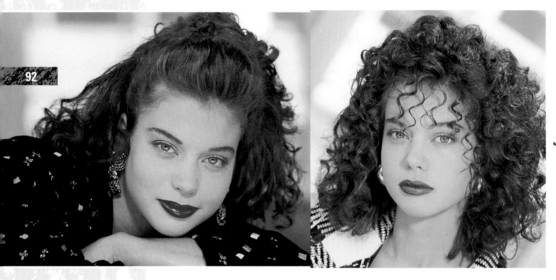

far left **Permed locks are clipped up on crown.**

left **The same locks worn loose and free. By Ellis Helen for Clairol Professional.**

right **Naturally curly hair is dried with a diffuser.**

far right **The curls are tamed slightly using wax. By Kathleen Bray for Clairol.**

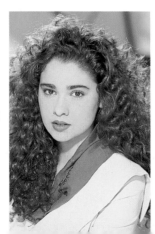

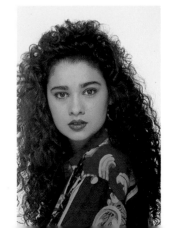

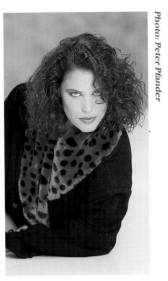

Photo: Peter Pfander

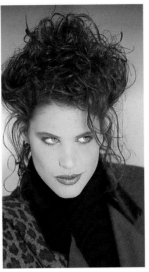

far left Curly hair is scrunch-dried with mousse.

left It is swept up for a more sophisticated look. By Stephen Wake at Level for Schwarzkopf.

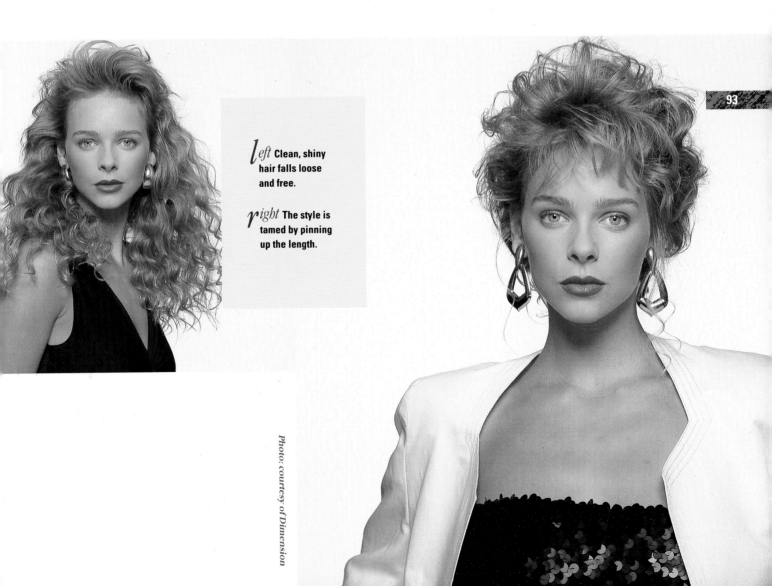

left Clean, shiny hair falls loose and free.

right The style is tamed by pinning up the length.

Photo: courtesy of Dimension

94

above **A soft ponytail is clasped to one side.**

left **The hair is worn long and loose.**

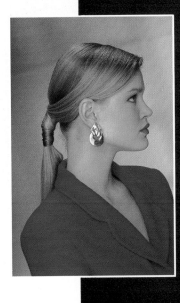

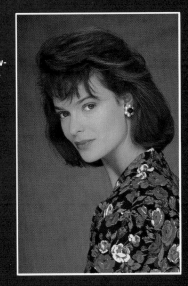

left Colour enhanced hair is worn in a covered ponytail.

below Both styles 'au naturelle'. By Kathleen Bray for Clairol.

right It is blow-dried back for movement.

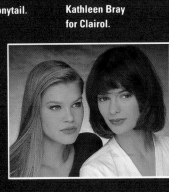

Photo: courtesy of Vendome Jewellery

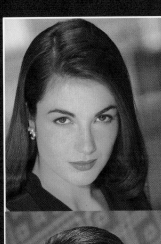

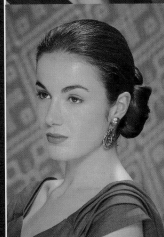

left A 'wash-in' 'wash-out' colour gives sheen to this loose style.

below The hair is clasped back into a soft bun at the nape for evening wear. By Kathleen Bray for Clairol.

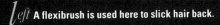

95

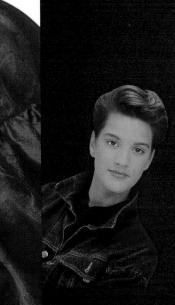

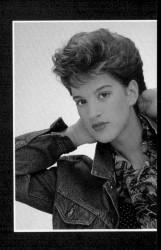

left A flexibrush is used here to slick hair back.

far right A more textured finish is achieved using mousse and drying upwards. By Keith Harris for Clairol.

below **Coloured with a semi-permanent brown and blow-dried back.**

far below **A golden rinse gives lights when hair is dressed high and curly. By Joel O'Sullivan for Clairol.**

below **Warm brown hair is blow-dried forward.**

far below **The natural curl is enhanced by using a pomade. By Stephen Wake at Level for Schwarzkopf.**

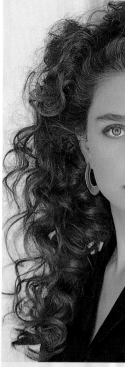

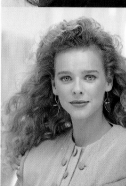

above **These styles show how bendy rollers can be used to create wild or more tamed curls. By Keith Harris for Clairol.**

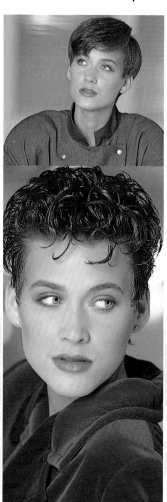

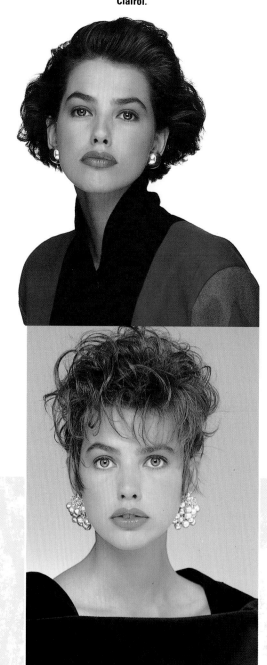

Photo: Peter Pfander

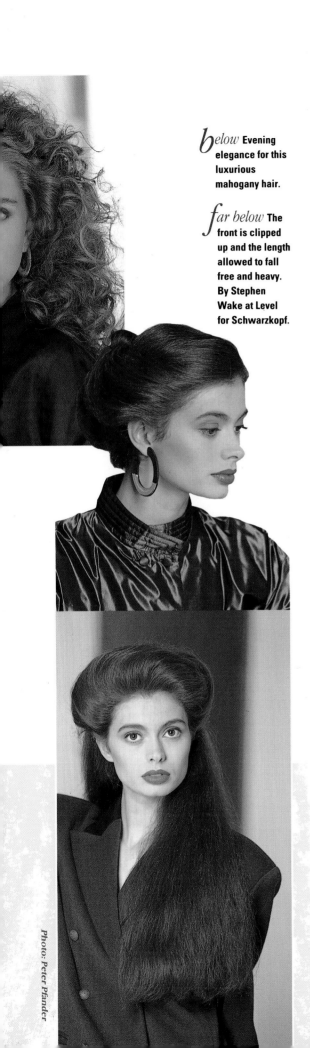

*b*elow Evening elegance for this luxurious mahogany hair.

*f*ar below The front is clipped up and the length allowed to fall free and heavy. By Stephen Wake at Level for Schwarzkopf.

Photo: Peter Pfander

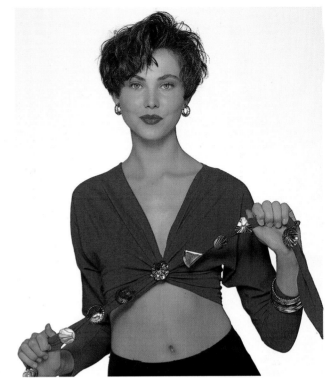

*a*bove The hair is blow-dried up and back.

*r*ight A vent brush and nozzle on the dryer gives a sophisticated finish.

*b*elow A neater result achieved using hairspray.

97

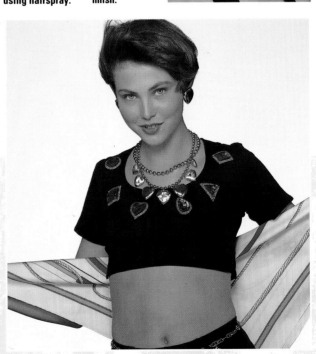

Photo: courtesy of Corocraft Jewellery.

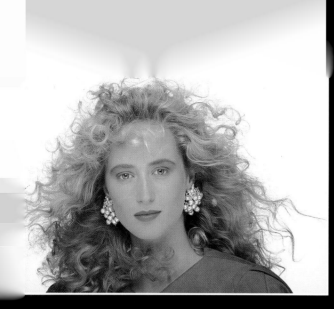

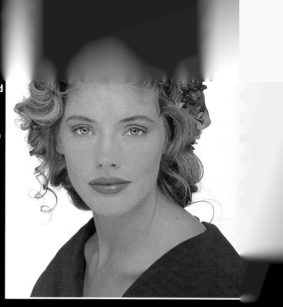

*l*eft Wild, tousled tresses.

*r*ight Tamed into a soft roll at the back. By Joel O'Sullivan for Clairol.

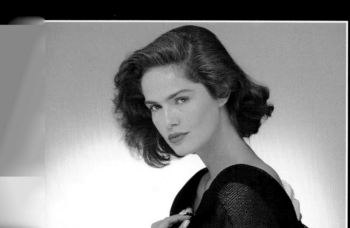

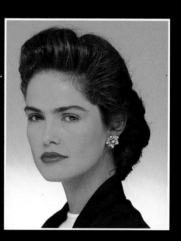

*l*eft A shoulder length bob is given a semi-permanent rinse.

*r*ight It is swept into an elegant, smooth design. By Joel O'Sullivan for Clairol.

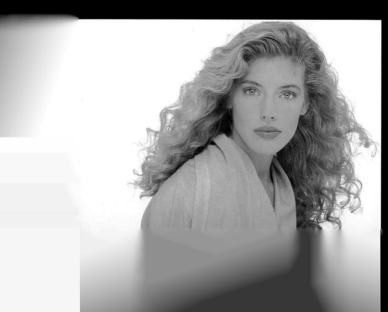

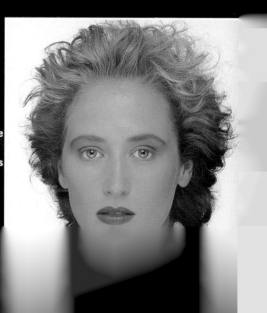

*l*eft A fresh, flowing strawberry blonde.

*r*ight Softly rolled at the back, leaving the front soft and allowing tendrils to fall. By Kathleen Bray for Clairol.

above **Stunning white-blonde hair is feathered on to the face.**

right **The hair is blow-dried close to the head for an alternative look. By Kathleen Bray for Clairol.**

Photo: Pete Underwood

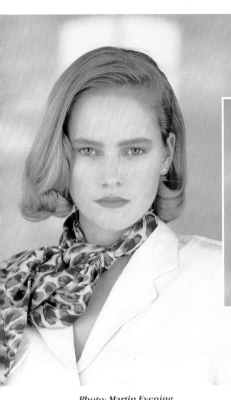

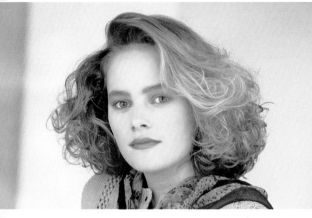

below Dried using the root massage technique.

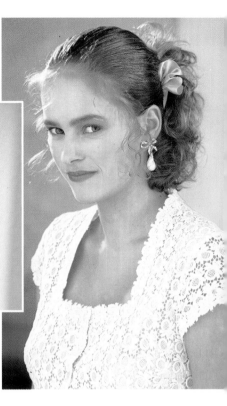

Mid-length hair is the most versatile. *left* Dried smooth and tipped under.

right Right: Teased into a curly ponytail. By Rebecca Cazaly for Wella.

Photo: Martin Evening

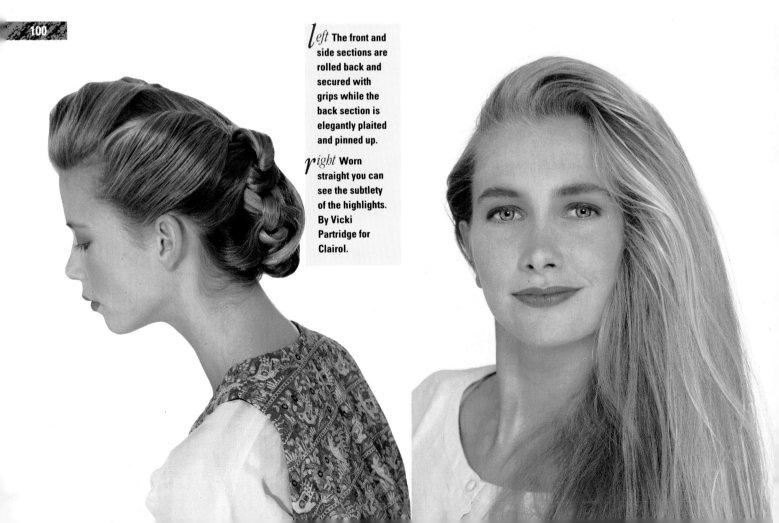

left The front and side sections are rolled back and secured with grips while the back section is elegantly plaited and pinned up.

right Worn straight you can see the subtlety of the highlights. By Vicki Partridge for Clairol.

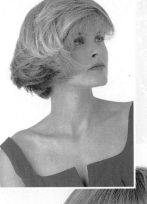

left The hair is bleached, tinted beige and dried to give root lift.

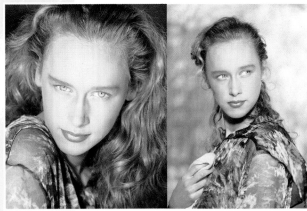

below left The hair is dried forwards into a polished cap. By Jeni for Clynol Hair.

Photo: Pete Underwood

Photo: Melissa Halstead

above Mousse is finger-woven through hair to give a waxed, textured look.

above right The top hair is dressed into a high ponytail. By Gary Hooker at Saks for Clynol Hair.

101

Long brown hair is given a deep mahogany glow and rich glossy sheen using a semi-permanent colour.

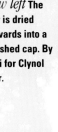

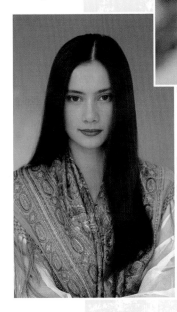

left A centre parted and loose style.

above The crown hair is dressed in a soft knot.

right The top hair is parted and rolled whilst length is curled. By Martin Unerman at Martin Gold for Wella.

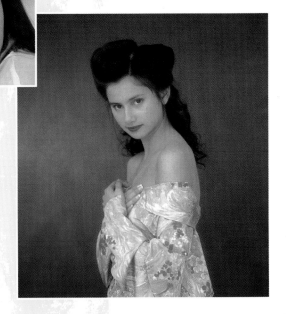

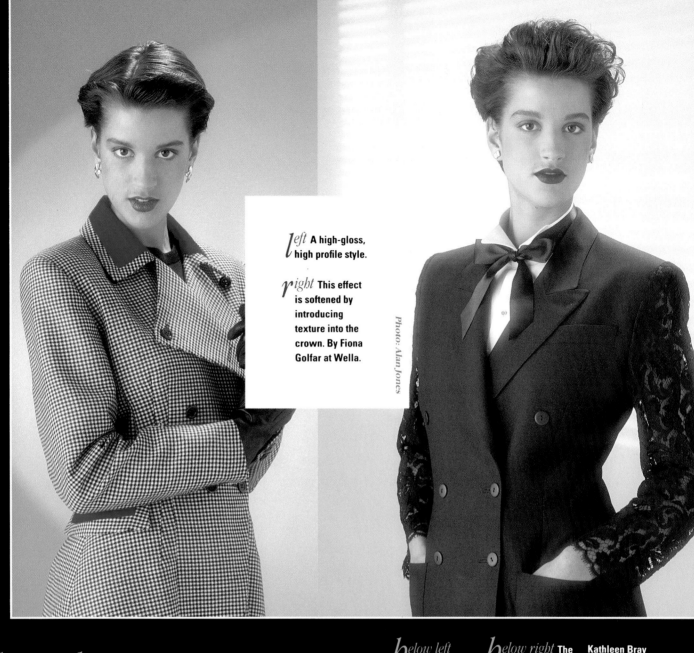

*l*eft A high-gloss, high profile style.

*r*ight This effect is softened by introducing texture into the crown. By Fiona Golfar at Wella.

Photo: Alan Jones

*b*elow left A simple twist transforms straight hair.

*b*elow right Towel-dried hair is gelled and wound into loose spiral curls which can be pinned up or left down for a more casual look. By Lisa Johansen at Macmillan.

*b*elow left Natural looking curls are easy with bendy rollers.

*b*elow right The same curls are softly clipped up allowing tendrils to fall loosely. By Kathleen Bray for Clairol.

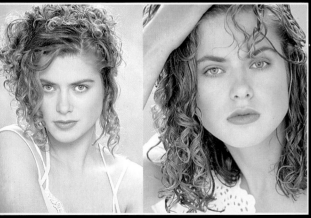

Photo: Ursula Steiger

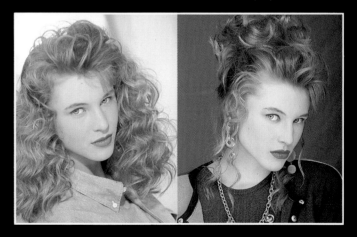

right The hair is set on heated rollers.

below Casual feminine curls are lightly pinned in place. By Keith Harris for Clairol.

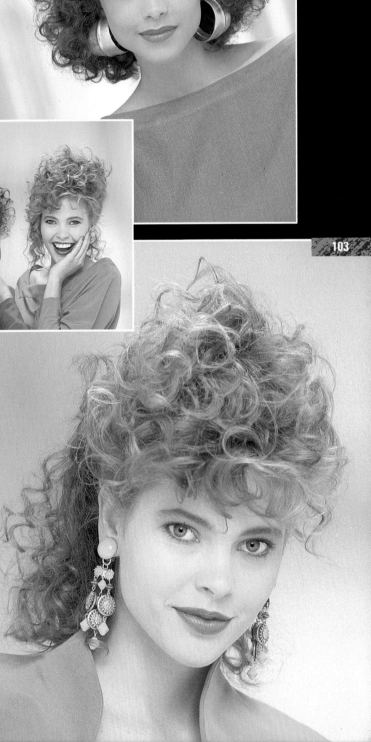

below Curls are secured with decorative slides.

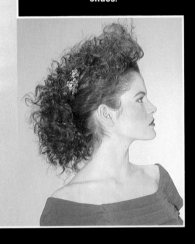

103

below A full and natural look. By Keith Harris for Clairol.

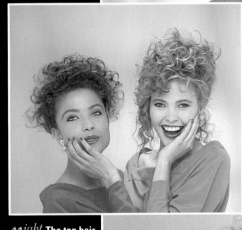

right The top hair is piled high and full, whilst the back cascades in curls. By Keith Harris for Clairol.

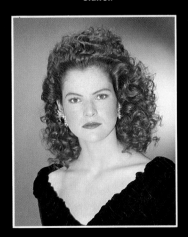

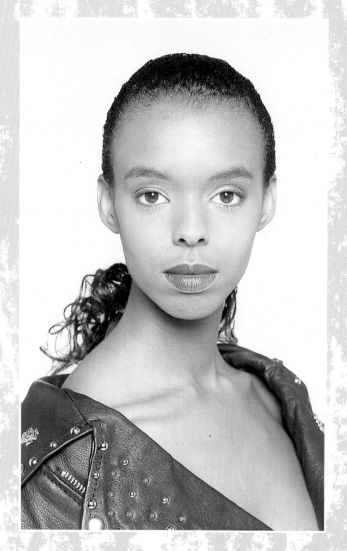

Black hair is scraped back and clasped into a ponytail at the nape. By Ellis Helen.

Black styles

Negroid hair has a unique texture. At first glance it appears thick and strong but this is deceptive. There are fewer hairs per square inch than any other type of hair so it rarely grows very thick. Also, the curved follicles give each hair a spring-like action which makes the curls appear short. The type and degree of curl is, in fact, the main difference between Caucasian and Black hair. Instead of growing and curling in a uniform manner the hair grows in various directions, thus making it fall in uneven frizzy waves. In addition, far from being strong, this type of hair is the weakest – fragile and dry, it rapidly loses moisture and needs daily moisturizing to keep it in condition.

In the past oils and grease were used to combat dryness and to protect the hair. The weight and heaviness of these products also clogged the hair follicles and sometimes led to hair loss. Strong detergent shampoos were often used which led to further problems of dryness and flaking scalps.

Today, specialist manufacturers provide preparations that are lighter and more easily absorbed into the hair. If you have Black hair it is important to take extra special care. As a guide you should always use a mild shampoo and conditioner each time you wash. If your hair has been chemically treated you should use a hot oil treatment at least every two weeks. Each day use a light film of moisturizing spray. Black hair is very dry and porous and will literally soak up any moisture in the atmosphere. When this happens the hair reverts back to its pre-styled state. Products called 'reversion resistant' sprays are designed to seal the hair shafts and prevent this happening.

A popular way of dressing Black hair is to straighten or 'relax' it. New products enable hairdressers to get the desired straighter hair with just a foundation of curl, to provide lift to the hair and enable the style to be dressed in a variety of ways. As this type of hair is so fragile I would strongly recommend

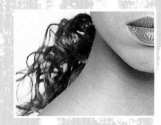

professional application of relaxing hair products at a salon that specializes in this technique. Colour can look stunning on Black hair and you can do this yourself using the wide variety of spray-on colours or glitter sprays which look superb on dark curls. If you want a colour rinse or lowlights, try coppery-gold shades – sheer magic! Bleaching is a very drastic process for Black hair and needs perfect maintainance, so, once again it is best left to the hairdresser.

Traditionally Black hair was plaited in classical corn-rows and this look is still popular today. The addition of coloured beads and ribbons will enhance this type of styling even further.

Here we show a beautiful selection of creations incorporating loops, ringlets and curls . . . .

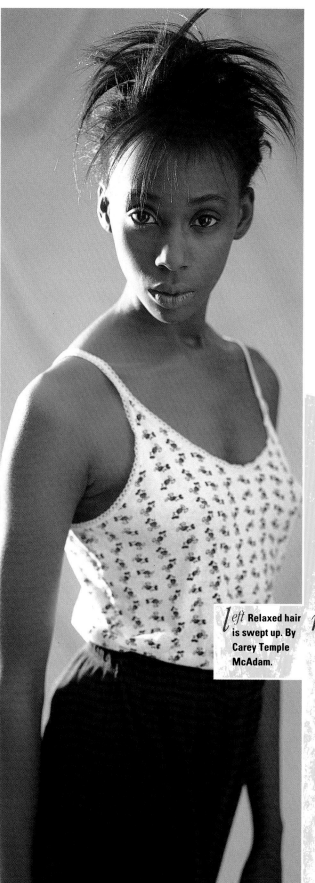

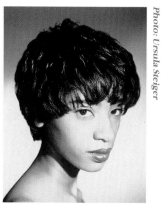

right The hair is layered and cut in a forward movement. By Lisa Johansen at Macmillan.

Photo: Ursula Steiger

left Relaxed hair is swept up. By Carey Temple McAdam.

right Black hair is bleached and razor cut. By Franklin Massahood at Morris Masterclass.

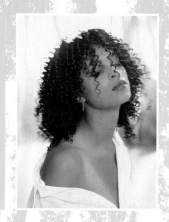

right Soft, spiral curls make this an easy-to-wear look. By Fields.

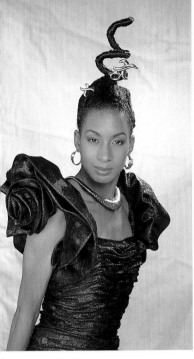

right This dramatic design is blow-dried. By Franklin Massahood at Morris Masterclass for Carson Products.

left A wired hair-piece helps create this style. By Splinters.

below The hair is relaxed and dressed with mousse. By Franklin Massahood at Morris Masterclass.

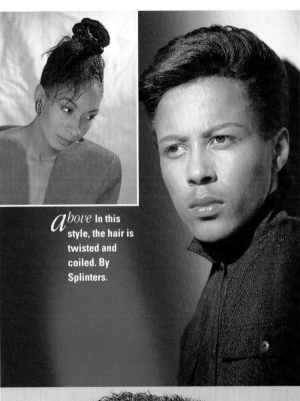

above In this style, the hair is twisted and coiled. By Splinters.

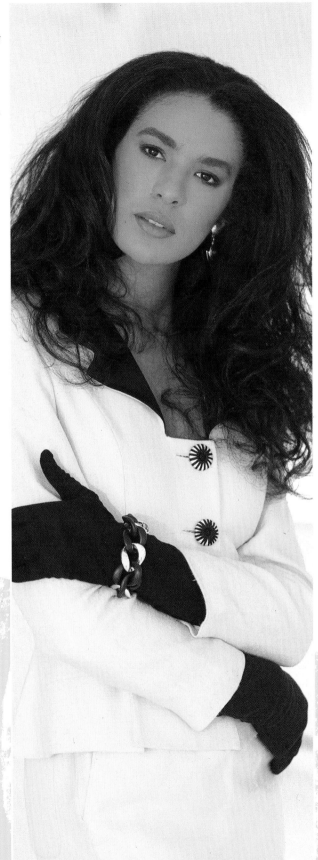

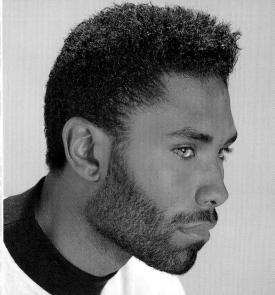

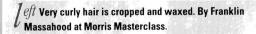

left Very curly hair is cropped and waxed. By Franklin Massahood at Morris Masterclass.

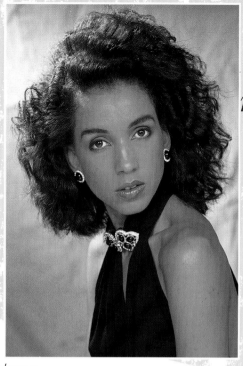

right **Mousse was applied to naturally curly hair which was then finger-dried, pressing waves into the front and building weight to the crown. By Gary Hooker at Saks for Clynol Hair.**

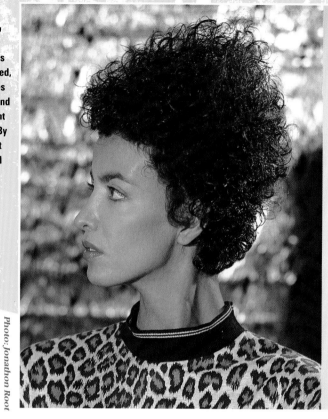

Photo: Jonathon Root

above **Finger-waves at the front add interest. By Splinters.**

below **Gold clips add an unusual touch to this style. By Errol Douglas at Edmonds for Schwarzkopf.**

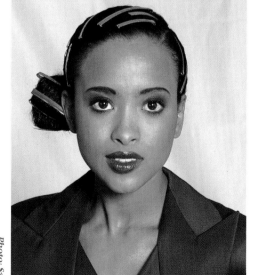

Photo: Sandro Hyams

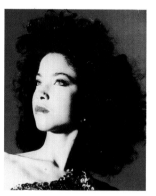

left **A mane of luxuriant curls. By Fields.**

right **The hair is twisted into a bun and the ends are fanned out and sprayed with fixing gel. By Franklin Massahood at Morris Masterclass for Carson Products.**

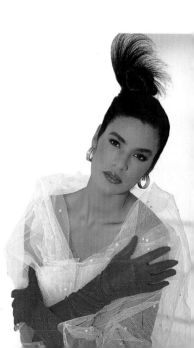

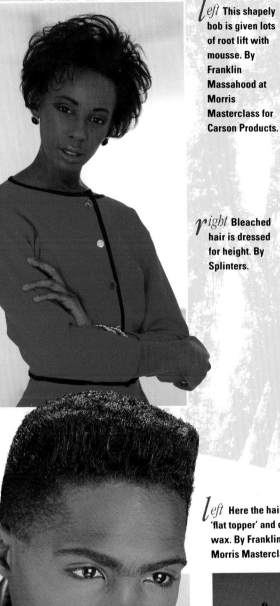

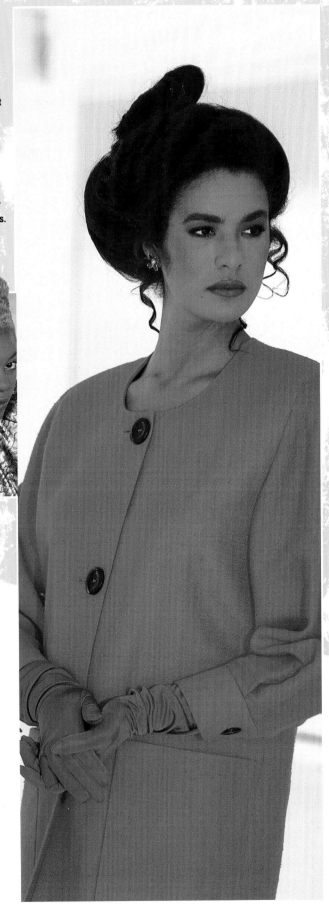

left This shapely bob is given lots of root lift with mousse. By Franklin Massahood at Morris Masterclass for Carson Products.

right An elegant bouffant bun with side tendrils. By Franklin Massahood at Morris Masterclass for Carson Products.

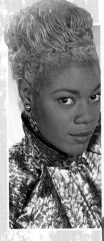

right Bleached hair is dressed for height. By Splinters.

109

left Here the hair is cut with a 'flat topper' and dressed with wax. By Franklin Massahood at Morris Masterclass.

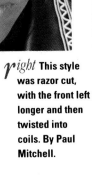

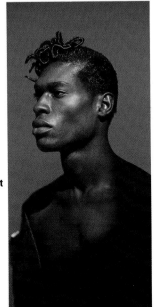

right This style was razor cut, with the front left longer and then twisted into coils. By Paul Mitchell.

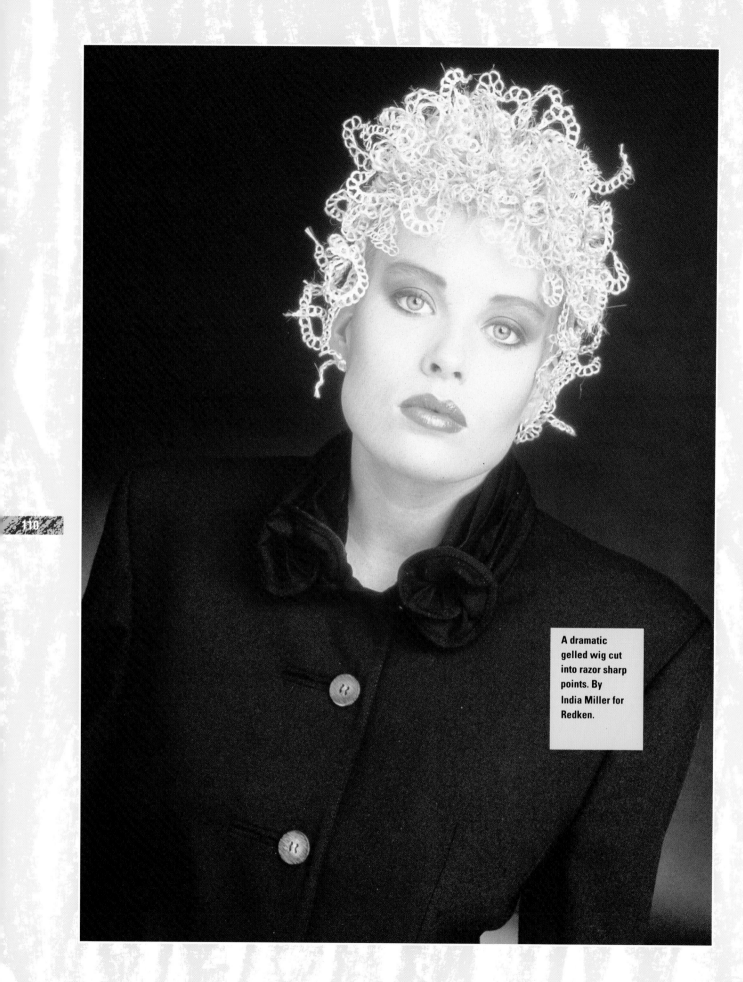

A dramatic
gelled wig cut
into razor sharp
points. By
India Miller for
Redken.

Wigs, extensions and hairpieces

In ancient Egypt wigs were worn by men and women on top of their natural hair. As hygiene became a consideration it was quite normal to shave the entire head and wear a wig! Many of these first styles were the immaculate wedge shapes recreated so well in the film, 'Cleopatra'. Later, vertical rows of separate curls also became popular.

Over the centuries the wearing of wigs has fluctuated in popularity. It was reported that Elizabeth I had more than 80 wigs. In the late sixteenth century the wig became a symbol of power and professionals – lawyers, doctors, judges and clergymen – wore them as a symbol of their status.

Wigs reached their most extravagant during the late seventeenth century with musical boxes, ornaments and even singing birds intertwined with the hair.

The French Revolution saw the decline of the wig and the change to more natural hair. By 1800 it was estimated that only one hundred and fifty thousand wig-wearers were left in Britain. The Incorporated Guild of Hairdressers, Wigmakers and Perfumiers was founded in 1882 to meet and promote the improvement of the social position and general welfare of its members. This august body still exists today.

Hairpieces or 'postiches' made a dramatic comeback in the 1960s. The advent of artificial fibres made it possible to mass produce wigs and pieces so that every woman could change her hairstyle in minutes. Sadly for the wigmakers, the meteoric rise in their trade was halted by Vidal Sassoon's cut and blow-dry.

Nowadays wigs and hairpieces are generally used to create exotic evening and fantasy designs to show off the hairdressers' skills, rather than worn by the general public. Wigs are still used extensively in TV commercials and films to help create character parts.

A revolutionary development of the last decade is hair extensions or dreadlocks. Developed by Simon Forbes of Antenna, hair extensions consist of Monofibre, braided into the hair and heat sealed for permanency. Extensions give instant length and can transform a short cut into long luxuriant locks in a matter of hours.

Worn by pop and film stars this innovation has been one of the most exciting in post-punk Britain. There is no limit to the type of styles that can be created by the use of extensions. They can be very natural-looking or free and funky. Once attached, extensions require no special after-care and can be left in for up to three months. Extensions can also be used to create shorter, more sophisticated styles. Curl, cut and colour can be added.

The styles shown on the following pages show hairdressing skills at their most visionary. Stunning creativity at its best – use the pictures to inspire you to experiment with a completely new appearance next time you want to make a grand entrance.

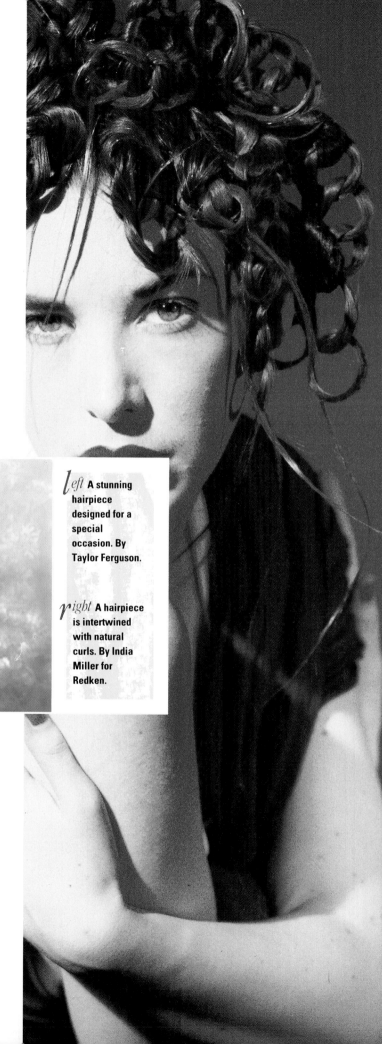

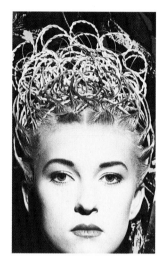

left An exotic
fantasy of
looped hair and
a 'crown' of
coils. By India
Miller for
Redken.

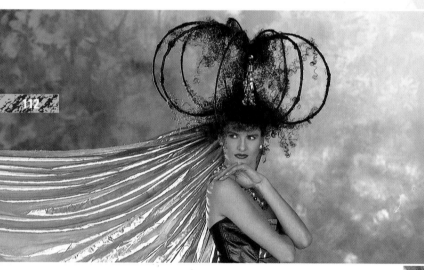

112

left A stunning
hairpiece
designed for a
special
occasion. By
Taylor Ferguson.

right A hairpiece
is intertwined
with natural
curls. By India
Miller for
Redken.

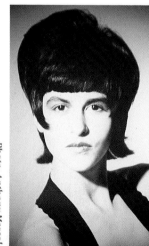

left This wig has
been cut into a
dramatic bob
shape. By Toni &
Guy.

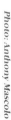

Photo: Anthony Mascolo

Photo: Bill Ling

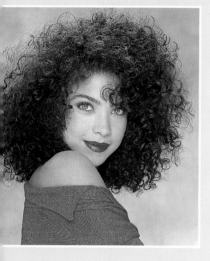

right **This hairpiece has been finely crocheted for a really unusual texture. By India Miller for Redken.**

left **A full wig is cut into a long graduated shape with the weigh retained round the back. By Beverly Kyprianou at Cobella for Schwarzkopf.**

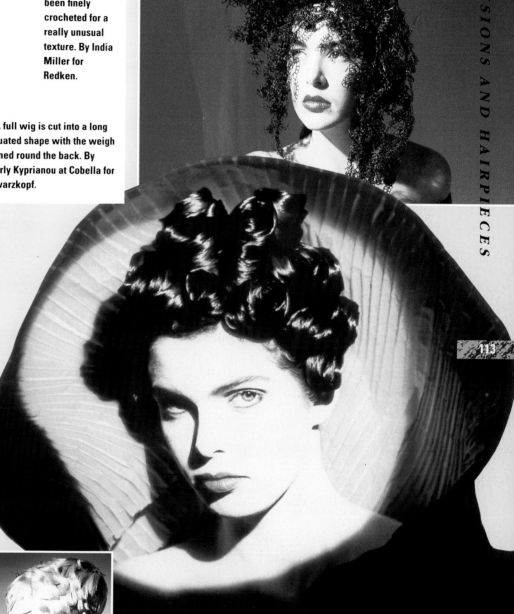

right **Glossy looped curls for the ultra-sophisticated lady. By Jason Miller for Redken.**

right **A blunt cut 60s style bouffant wig. By Toni & Guy.**

Photo: Anthony Mascolo

113

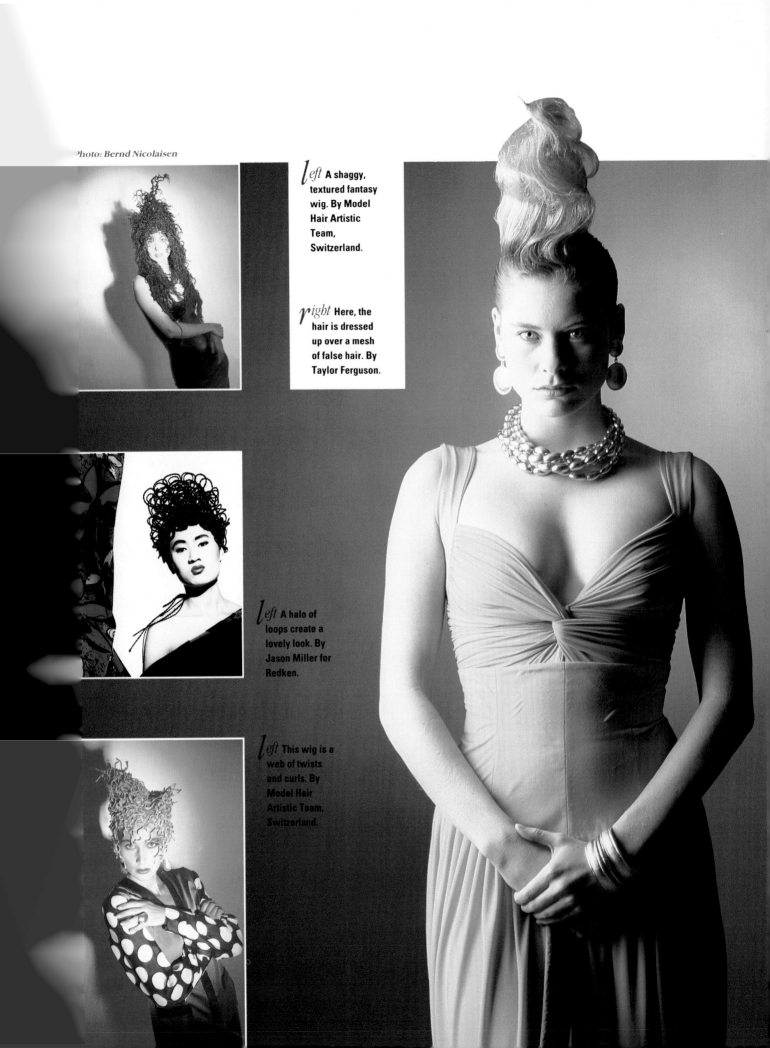

Photo: Bernd Nicolaisen

left **A shaggy, textured fantasy wig. By Model Hair Artistic Team, Switzerland.**

right **Here, the hair is dressed up over a mesh of false hair. By Taylor Ferguson.**

left **A halo of loops create a lovely look. By Jason Miller for Redken.**

left **This wig is a web of twists and curls. By Model Hair Artistic Team, Switzerland.**

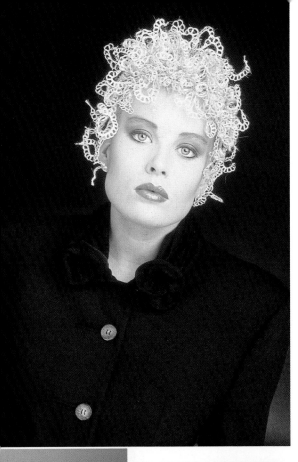

left Delicate crocheted extensions. By India Miller for Redken.

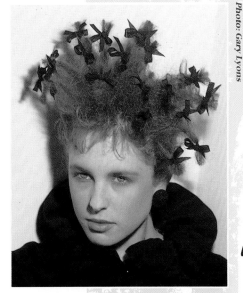

Photo: Gary Lyons

left Extensions are dressed with styling spray and ribbons. By Jeanne Braa for Paul Mitchell.

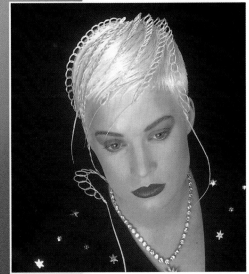

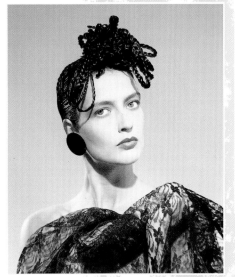

left A mass of fine plaits are woven into this intricate creation. By Taylor Ferguson.

115

above Individual crocheted extensions add a second dimension to this classic short cut. By India Miller for Redken.

right Black hair, twisted and gelled. By Paul Mitchell.

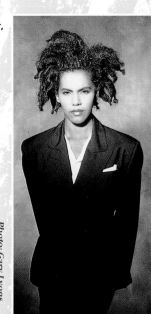

Photo: Gary Lyons

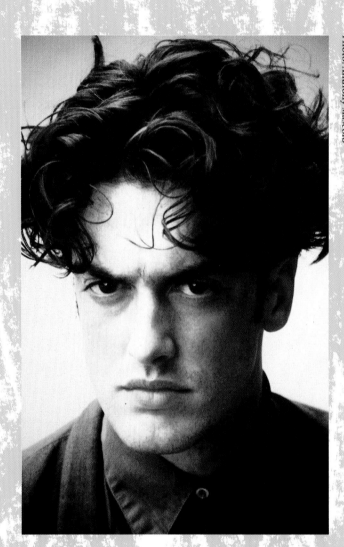

This ruffled, layered cut is dressed with mousse. By Tony & Guy.

Photo: Anthony Mascolo

116

Men's styles

The fundamentals of hairdressing as a profession lie in the art of barbering and the razor. As early as the Egyptian period the first roughly hewn razors appeared and there are many myths surrounding the wearing of the beard. It is said that during the time of Alexander the Great his troops were instructed to shave off their beards so that the opposition would not be able to grab them!

Barbers were also surgeons and dentists. In England, the Worshipful Company of Barbers and Surgeons was formed in 1307 and still exists with magnificient headquarters in the City of London.

Over the centuries men have dressed their beards and moustaches in every conceivable way: powdered, waxed, dried, curled, trimmed, straightened and preened to perfection as dictated by the fashion of the day.

The widespread wearing of wigs by men came about during the late sixteenth century. The problem of cleanliness prompted this action to a certain extent. Men would have the wigs made from their own hair and periodically return them to the barber for de-lousing, re-curling and powdering. Men engaged in what were termed gentile professions wore wigs and this tradition still holds today in legal circles.

Short back and sides and clean-shaven faces became popular during the First World War and this look persisted until the 60s. In this new age of freedom men grew their hair into Beatle crops and the emergence of the hippies heralded long flowing, unkempt hair.

The existence of traditional barbers was threatened with men demanding the same standard of cutting and styling as women. The birth of the unisex salon heralded a minor revolution in hairdressing circles. Recently areas for men's and women's styling have become more segregated and there is a return to the traditional barber's shops. However, these new premises have a much more upmarket ambience and there is very little price differential between these and women's salons.

Styling aids have made a tremendous difference to the grooming of men's hair. Products are designed specifically for the male market and it has become acceptable for mousses and gels to be used as part of a daily routine.

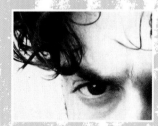

There is still resistance to perms and colour for men with research figures showing that an average of only 8 per cent of men risk a colour change and only 4 per cent try a perm! However, milder perms which create root lift, body and volume without curls are coming on to the market. It is probably only a matter of time before men realize that this technique can give limp hair added volume and thickness and make unruly, heavy hair more easily controlled.

Overleaf you will see some slick styles for men – all groomed to perfection.

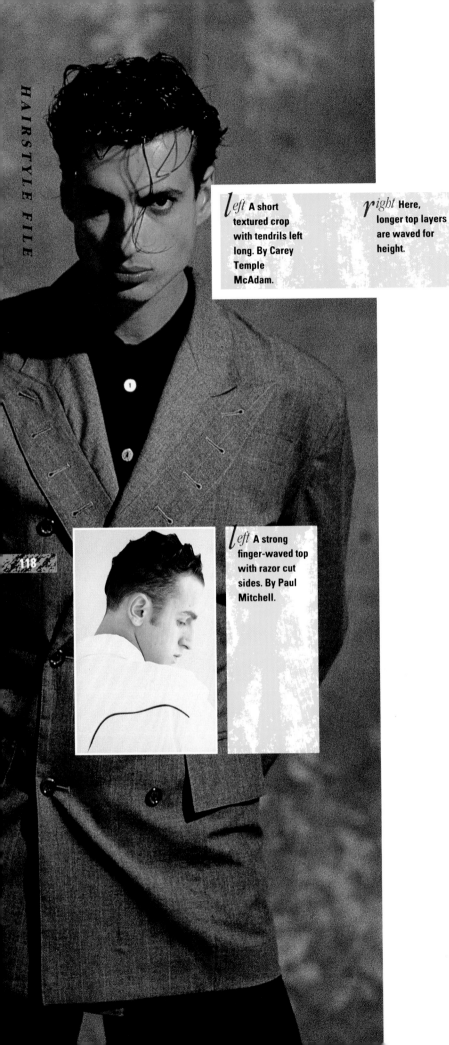

left A short textured crop with tendrils left long. By Carey Temple McAdam.

right Here, longer top layers are waved for height.

left A strong finger-waved top with razor cut sides. By Paul Mitchell.

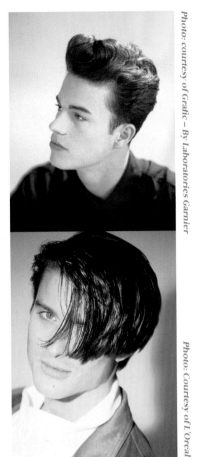

Photo: courtesy of Grafic – By Laboratoires Garnier

Photo: Courtesy of L'Oreal

above This longer-look style is modelled into shape with wet look gel.

below Blonde highlights give this cut definition. By Model Hair, Switzerland.

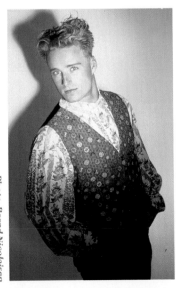

Photo: Bernd Nicolaisen

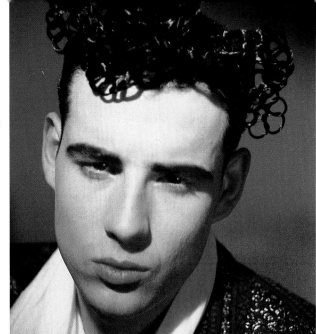

right This style consists of shaved sides with extensions looped on the crown. By India Miller for Schwarzkopf.

left The hair is permed then styled with foam. By Jeni for Clynol Hair.

Photo: Pete Underwood

right This hair is swept upwards using strong gel and mousse. By Paul Mitchell.

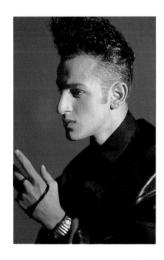

119

left Here the hair is cut close into the nape and left longer on top to take advantage of its natural wave. By Taylor Ferguson.

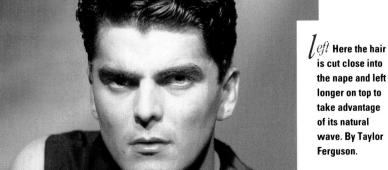

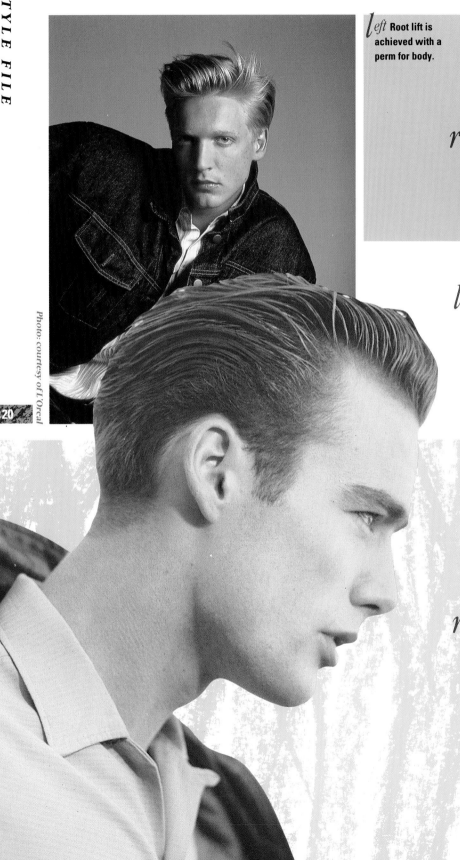

Photo: courtesy of L'Oreal

120

left **Root lift is achieved with a perm for body.**

right **Naturally thick, slightly wavy hair is moussed and styled forward. By Melvyn & Friends.**

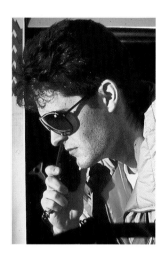

left **A strong, rugged outdoor look. By Paul Mitchell.**

right **Shorter length, layered hair has been heavily waxed to create height and emphasize the casual texture. By Model Hair, Switzerland.**

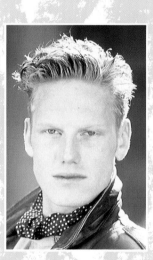

Photo: Bernd Nicolaisen

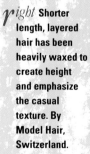

below **This 50s crop is blow-dried straight.**

right **Natural curls are given a textured look with forming spray. By Richard Dalton at Claridges for Clairol Professional.**

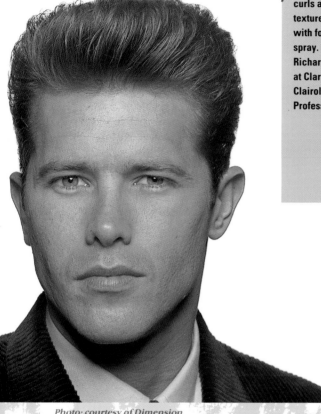

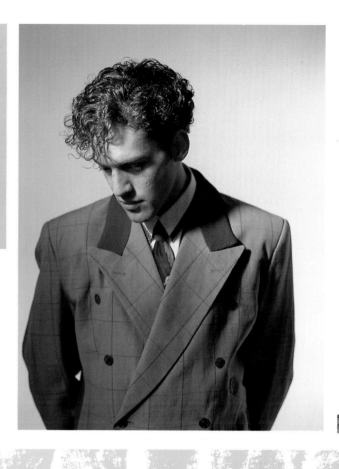

Photo: courtesy of Dimension

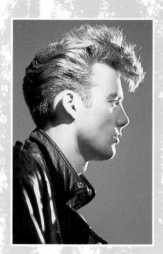

left **A teddy-boy style with front quiff. By Paul Mitchell.**

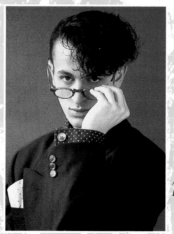

right **Wet-look gel creates this mean and moody look.**

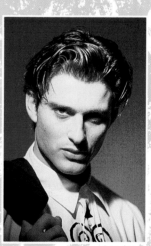

above **Slicked back and sides with long textured front. By Paul Mitchell.**

Photo: courtesy of L'Oreal

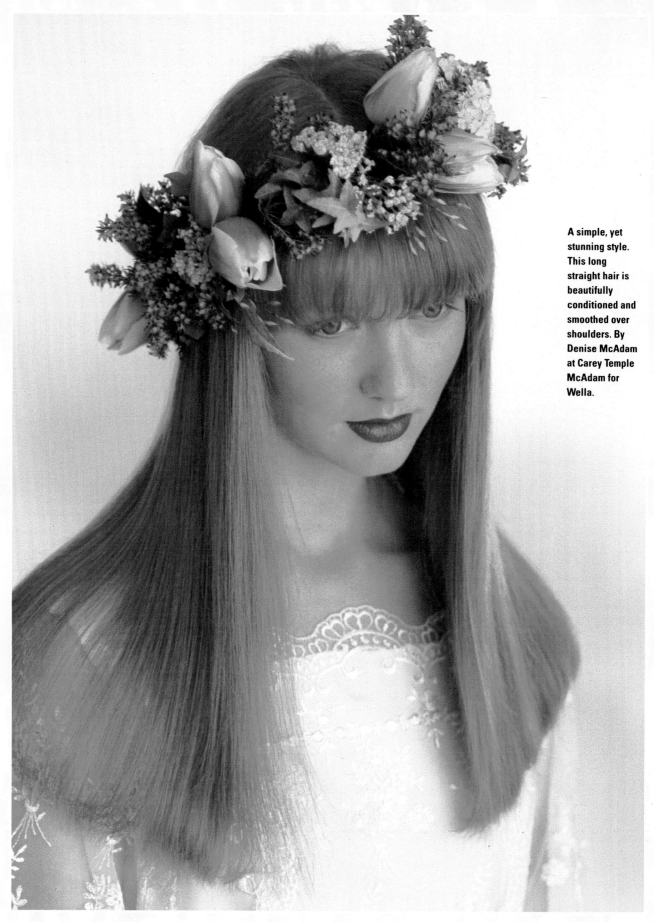

Photo: Bill Morton

A simple, yet stunning style. This long straight hair is beautifully conditioned and smoothed over shoulders. By Denise McAdam at Carey Temple McAdam for Wella.

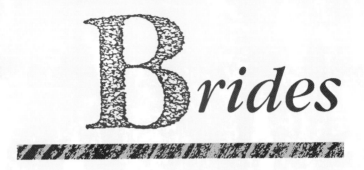

Brides

Traditionally brides have always adorned their hair with heavy braids, ribbons and hairpieces, but

surprisingly the fashion for white gowns only came into being in the middle of the eighteenth century. Until this time the bride always wore black!

The essence of a successful bridal hairstyle is one that will look stunning throughout the entire wedding day. In order to achieve this forward planning is required.

Firstly, remember that your hair is going to be the focal point and you should make sure it is in perfect condition. Treat yourself to a series of intensive conditioning treatments. These can be done at home or in a salon, but should start at least eight weeks before the wedding.

Next, if you intend having your hair done by a hairdresser on your wedding day – don't make that your one and only visit. Consult the hairdresser prior to the wedding and discuss your chosen style. Take your head-dress or veil to

the salon plus a sketch of the dress that illustrates the neckline details and if possible a swatch of fabric. Then you can work together to choose the perfect look. Remember that the key to a successful bride is simplicity. A heavily lacquered and back-combed creation may look good going up the aisle, but what will it look like when you change into your going away outfit? A natural, soft style that is caught up loosely for the ceremony and then allowed to fall free later is ideal. If you decide on a perm, four weeks before the 'big day' is the time to have it, as this enables the curls to settle down, and gives you time to learn how to handle the new texture. If your hair is long you could try a romantic and natural looking spiral perm or if your hair is shorter maybe you will just need a body perm for lift and bounce. If you want a curly look without a perm try using heated bendy rollers.

Two weeks to go and it's time to get your hair trimmed and make sure that your hair colour is looking good. If you intend to have any high or

lowlights, have them now!

One week – now is the time to check your appointment for the morning of the wedding and have a trial-run of the chosen style.

If you follow this suggested routine you can be sure that by your wedding day your hair will be in tip-top condition and ready for styling to the look of your dreams.

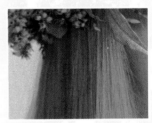

Bridal hair designs can incorporate a beautiful array of accessories. Circlets of flowers, braids bound with ribbons, strands of white pearls or traditional tiaras – the choice is yours.

The bridal styles featured overleaf show a softness and femininity that is a joy to behold.

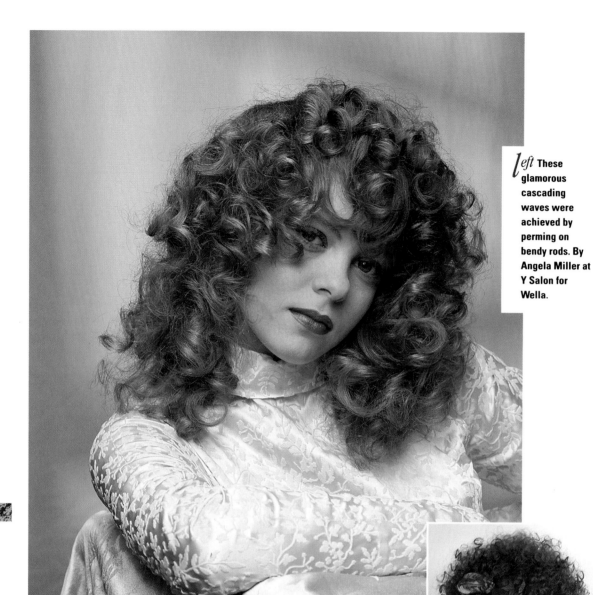

*l*eft These glamorous cascading waves were achieved by perming on bendy rods. By Angela Miller at Y Salon for Wella.

*l*eft These romantic, ruffled curls are held in place by hairspray. By Denise McAdam at Carey Temple McAdam for Wella.

Photo: Bill Morton

*l*eft This permed hair was treated with a texturizing styling mousse to create profuse waves.

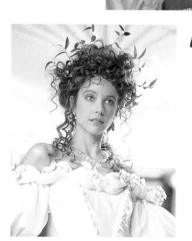

*l*eft A mass of upswept curls with tiny ringlets. By Andrew Collinge.

Photo: courtesy of L'Oreal

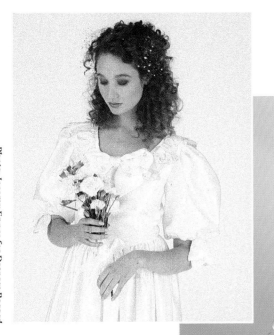

Photo: Jeremy Ennes for Drapers Record

above **Small curls and ringlets are intertwined with flowers. By Kriss Hass at Partners.**

right **Sections of hair are caught at the back for this sleek style. By Taylor Ferguson.**

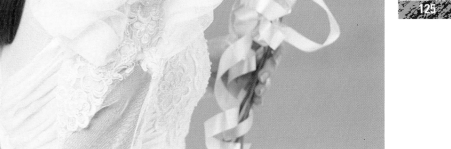

125

right **This long hair is dressed into an unusual chignon at the nape of the neck. By Denise McAdam at Carey, Temple McAdam.**

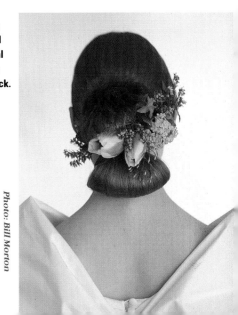

above **A beautifully soft and feminine style topped with white roses. By Andrew Collinge.**

right **An elegant topknot encircled by a tiara. By Jo Seward at Carey Temple McAdam for Wella.**

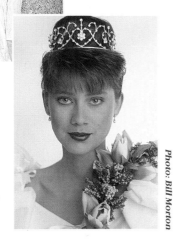

Photo: Bill Morton

Photo: Bill Morton

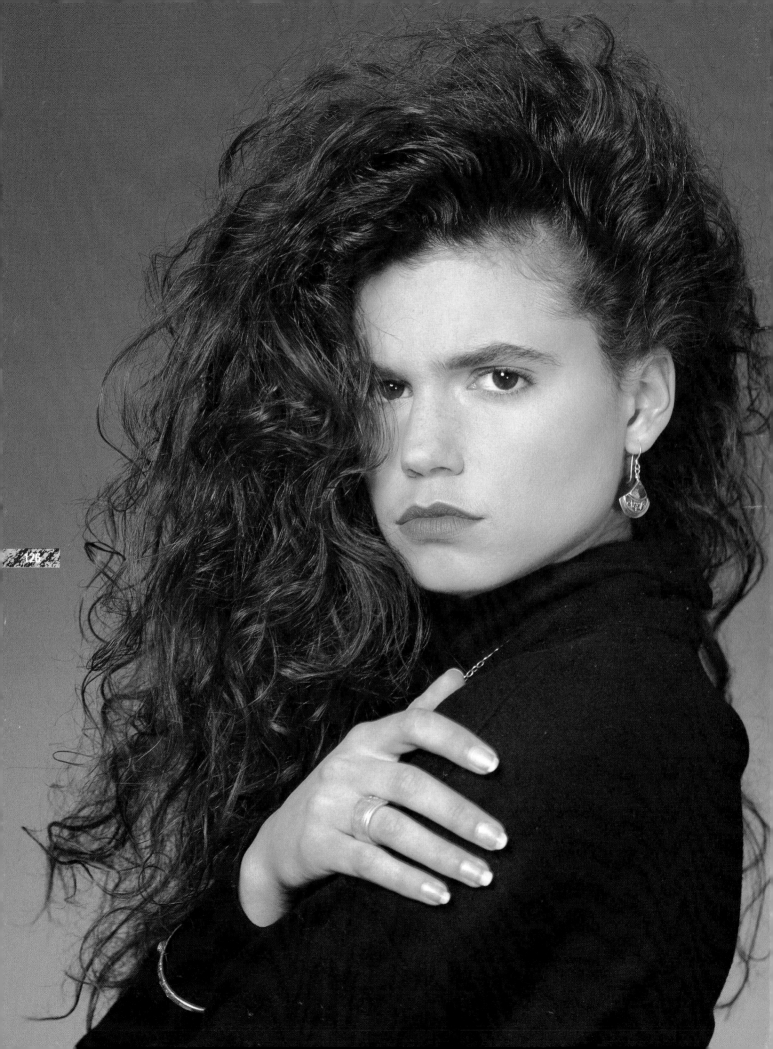

Acknowledgements

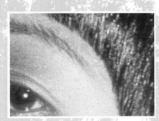

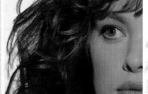

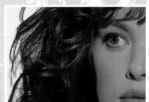

Chazz Balkwill at Donato, Canada
Karen Berman Associates Ltd
Norman Bloomfield
Roberta Brown
Chris Burridge at Tresemme
Judy Burton at Vivienne Tomei PR Ltd
Felicity Calthorpe Associates
JC
Alison Chesterton at Palm Springs
John Claughton and Angela Rae at Wella
Andrew Collinge
Hazel Collins at Ellis Helen
Debra Leggoe at Concept PR
Christopher Dove
Ian Duncan
Shirley Dunmall
Annabel Eker and Kate Goodman at Maureen Cropper Associates
Anne Ferguson
Felicity Forbes
Kate Friis and Louise Wood at Kate Friis PR
Andrea Goodenough at Rogol Goodkind Associates
Catherine Graham and Liz Hindmarsh at Liz Hindmarsh PR
Keith Harris, Freelancers
Robert Heed
Guy Kremer
Harold Leighton and Leslie Spears at Paul Mitchell and 365
(with special thanks to *Eamonn McCabe; Kim Knott; Russ Malkin; John Austin; Ursula Steiger; Gary Lyons and Tony Moussoulides*).
Pat Mascolo at Toni & Guy
Franklin Massahood at Morris Masterclass
Angela Miller
Charlie Miller
Helen Oppenheim, New York
Derek Pace
Cathy A Schoedes, Bumble & Bumble, New York
Karin Silverstein at Carol Hayes Associates
Karen Stainer
Rachael Vining and Liz Felhofer at L'Oreal
Stephen Wake at Level
Margot Walton-Clark

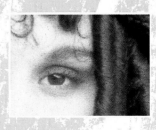

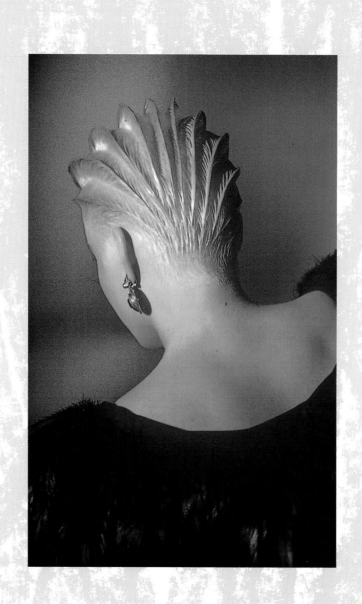

Guildford College
Learning Resource Centre
Please return on or before the last date shown.
No further issues or renewals if any items are overdue.
"7 Day" loans are **NOT** renewable.

08 SEP 2003

2 1 OCT 2003

-7 JUN 2006

2 9 NOV 2006

3 0 MAY 2012

Class: 646.724 WAD

Title: Hairstyle file.

Author: WADESON, Jacki

WITHDRAWN

106229